Pocket Guide to Teaching for Clinical Instructors

Pocket Guide to Teaching for Clinical Instructors

Advanced Life Support Group
Resuscitation Council UK

FOURTH EDITION

Edited by

Kate Denning
Lead Educator for ALSG

and

Alan Charters
Clinical Lead for ALSG

Kevin Mackie
Lead Educator for RCUK

Andrew Lockey
Clinical Lead for RCUK

♡ **Resuscitation Council UK**

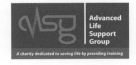

WILEY Blackwell

Contents

Working group

Mandy Brailsford MSc PGCE FHEA RN Head of Education, Contracts and Commissioning, Workforce, Training and Education Directorate, NHS England, North East and Yorkshire Region

Patricia Conaghan SFHEA FERC Senior Lecturer, Division of Nursing, Midwifery and Social Work, School of Health Sciences, Faculty of Biology, Medicine and Health, The University of Manchester, Manchester

Kate Denning PhD MA PGCE BA Director of Education and Development, Advanced Life Support Group; Honorary Lecturer, Keele University

Clare Duffy BA Director of Operations, Advanced Life Support Group, Manchester

Catriona Fleming MA BSc RN Education Lead Resuscitation Practitioner, Oxford University Hospitals NHS Foundation Trust

Paul Greig D.Phil MBChB PGCME MAcadeME BScMedSci FRCA Consultant Anaesthetist, Guy's and St Thomas' NHS Foundation Trust; Senior Clinical Research Fellow, Nuffield Department of Clinical Neurosciences, University of Oxford

Isabelle Hamilton-Bower MSc PGDipEd BSc Clinical Lead, Resuscitation Council UK, London

Alan Jervis MBA PGCME CMgr MCMI Head of Education, Cornwall Partnership NHS Foundation Trust, Education and Training Department, Cornwall

Joanna Lawrence MBA RN FHEA EQA Senior Coach Practitioner, Chief Executive Officer, Back to Life Limited

Kevin Mackie MSc PGDipEd BA Clinical Lead for
Education, RCUK; Honorary Lecturer, Keele University;
Consultant in Medical Education and Managing Director,
KCM Training Ltd, Peterborough

Nicki Morgan FRCEM Consultant in Emergency
Medicine, North Bristol NHS Trust

Josephine Octobre MSc BSc PGCert RN Rural and
Remote Emergency Nurse, New South Wales, Australia

Barry Smith MMedSci BA(PCE) Clinical Skills Lecturer
and Manager, Cambridge University Hospitals; Affiliated
Lecturer, School of Clinical Medicine, University of
Cambridge

Duncan Smith PhD MSc MN PGCert DTN RN FHEA
Senior Lecturer in Advanced Practice Nursing, City,
University of London; Honorary Consultant Nurse, Patient
Emergency Response and Resuscitation Team, University
College London Hospitals NHS Foundation Trust, London

Fiona Smith MSc PGCTLHE BSc RN Associate Dean for
Learning and Teaching, Faculty of Health Sciences and
Sport, University of Stirling

Contributors to the fourth edition

Mandy Brailsford MSc PGCE FHEA RN Head of Education, Contracts and Commissioning, Workforce, Training and Education Directorate, NHS England, North East and Yorkshire Region

Alan Charters DHealthSci MAEd PGDipEd BSc RSCN RGN Consultant Practitioner, Paediatric Emergency Care, Portsmouth, UK

Patricia Conaghan SFHEA FERC Senior Lecturer, Division of Nursing, Midwifery and Social Work, School of Health Sciences, Faculty of Biology, Medicine and Health, The University of Manchester, Manchester

Thomas Creten UK/ERC Educator Antwerp, Belgium

Jessica Denning BSc PGCE Assistant Producer BBC Education, Manchester

Kate Denning PhD MA PGCE BA Director of Education and Development, Advanced Life Support Group; Honorary Lecturer, Keele University

Catriona Fleming MA BSc RN Education Lead Resuscitation Practitioner, Oxford University Hospitals NHS Foundation Trust

Paul Greig D.Phil MBChB PGCME MAcadeME BScMedSci FRCA Consultant Anaesthetist, Guy's and St Thomas' NHS Foundation Trust; Senior Clinical Research Fellow, Nuffield Department of Clinical Neurosciences, University of Oxford

Alan Jervis MBA PGCME CMgr MCMI Head of Education, Cornwall Partnership NHS Foundation Trust, Education and Training Department, Cornwall

Joanna Lawrence MBA RN FHEA EQA Senior Coach Practitioner, Chief Executive Officer, Back to Life Limited

Andrew Lockey MBE PhD FRCS(A&E) FRCEM Consultant in Emergency Medicine, Calderdale and Huddersfield NHS Foundation Trust, Halifax; Visiting Professor in Emergency Medicine, University of Huddersfield; President of Resuscitation Council UK

Eleanor Mackie BA PGCE Primary Educator, Peterborough

Kevin Mackie MSc PGDipEd BA Clinical Lead for Education, RCUK; Honorary Lecturer, Keele University; Consultant in Medical Education and Managing Director KCM Training Ltd, Peterborough

Mary Mackie Author and playwright, Heacham, Norfolk

Nicki Morgan FRCEM Consultant in Emergency Medicine, North Bristol NHS Trust

Josephine Octobre MSc BSc PGCert RN Rural and Remote Emergency Nurse, New South Wales, Australia

Barry Smith MMedSci BA(PCE) Clinical Skills Lecturer and Manager, Cambridge University Hospitals; Affiliated Lecturer, School of Clinical Medicine, University of Cambridge

Duncan Smith PhD MSc MN PGCert DTN RN FHEA Senior Lecturer in Advanced Practice Nursing, City, University of London; Honorary Consultant Nurse, Patient Emergency Response and Resuscitation Team, University College London Hospitals NHS Foundation Trust. London

Fiona Smith MSc PGCTLHE BSc RN Associate Dean for Learning and Teaching, Faculty of Health Sciences and Sport, University of Stirling

Foreword

It is fascinating to see this fourth edition of the *Pocket Guide to Teaching for Clinical Instructors* (commonly known as the 'Blue Book') as an evolution of medical education, evolving alongside the experience and increasingly robust evidence base that underpins adult education.

It is worth taking a moment to consider the impact that this book has had since the first edition was written back in 1998 by medical educators engaged with the RCUK and the ALSG to support the Generic Instructor Courses (GIC). At that time the focus was on equipping educators to deliver the GIC, and it took a pragmatic approach to improve the learning experience of candidates through the education of the educators. I would also argue that the true educational impact of the Blue Book (and the GIC courses in general) has extended far beyond the life support courses they were designed for, and into the wider healthcare education setting. Nearly all of the instructors and candidates who attend our courses also work in clinical practice, and thus directly or indirectly treat patients. I frequently see educators use to good effect the techniques pioneered in the Blue Book in their practice, clearly demonstrating the widespread adoption of its principles.

This fourth edition embraces our understanding of how clinicians learn, and how that can be translated into practice. It is surprisingly rare to see educational texts that make the link between theory and advice in such a concise, practical and clear way, and this is perhaps the greatest achievement of this book. There is a subtle shift in this edition from specific instructional techniques to a more adaptable approach reflecting the current evidence base that advocates a more flexible and bespoke approach which brings learners and educators together. It is great looking back at how much has changed over four editions, reflecting changes in the wider educational context.

Although designed to support the GIC courses, the book is relevant to all involved in clinical education, can be read in a weekend, and will undoubtably improve the learning experience at a time when service pressures mean that every educational moment is precious. What is clear in the text, and also on the GIC courses, is that teaching and learning can be taught and improved. There is much to learn here and I would recommend this text to all involved in clinical education and not just those completing a GIC course. For current instructors the linkage of theory to practice is even closer in this edition and I will personally be using many of the techniques described, especially with regard to the careful use of language in small group facilitations. That, like many others, is a great example of how subtle changes from the educator can make really meaningful differences to the learner. The book is full of such examples and they are all worth revisiting.

In recent years there has been a much greater understanding of equality, diversity and inclusion in education, although there is still a long way to go in many settings. This edition provides guidance and a better understanding of issues such as neurodiversity (especially important in assessment settings) and increases our understanding of how to maintain standards, whilst also adapting to the variability, needs and challenges that our learners face. This is an area that I see developing over future editions and was especially pleased to see focused on here.

Ultimately, the aim of clinical education is to improve the care of patients. Learning and education are an essential component of high-quality care, and by improving the education and learning of thousands I have no doubt that the Blue Book has a remarkable legacy for educators, learners and patients.

Simon Carley
Consultant in Emergency Medicine and HEMS Consultant
Dean, Royal College of Emergency Medicine
Professor, Manchester Academic Health Sciences Centre,
University of Manchester
Creator and Senior Author, St Emlyn's Blog and Podcast

Preface to the fourth edition

Welcome to this fourth edition of what has become known as the 'Blue Book'. This edition has been extensively revised to reflect changes in the educational delivery of many provider courses. We have tried to simplify the academic language to make it more readable, applicable and accessible, and we hope the more modern style of the book will be engaging for our diverse range of readers.

There is some new content that reflects the nature of contemporary teaching and learning; with equality, diversity and inclusion and psychological safety being covered much more thoroughly than in previous editions.

As with previous editions the book is intended as an aid to reflection: something which you can, and hopefully will, consult on many occasions before, during and after your courses. It does not contain all the answers, but it will provide something against which you can test your experiences. You will not find a blueprint for teaching here, rather some thoughts about the basics which we hope you will adapt to your personality and creativity. In the end, of course, it is what works for you and your learners that matters.

If you have read any of the previous editions, you will find a change to some of the language used on the Generic Instructor Course. We use 'Prepare, Open, Facilitate, Close' throughout this edition as a framework for planning and facilitating learning and the book is much more about facilitating learning than teaching through instructional techniques.

We would like to thank all of the authors and contributors for their hard work in writing, refining and editing this edition. We also thank our instructors (new and old, local and international) for many fruitful conversations and for giving their time so freely to support our mutual aim of saving lives by providing training.

Kate Denning – Lead Educator for ALSG

Kevin Mackie – Lead Educator for RCUK

Alan Charters – Clinical Lead for ALSG

Andrew Lockey – Clinical Lead for RCUK

Acknowledgments and dedication

A great many people have put a lot of hard work into the production of this book, and the accompanying Generic Instructor Course (GIC). The editors would like to thank all the contributors for their efforts and all the GIC instructors who took the time to send us their comments on the earlier editions and for their continued hard work in delivering the course.

We would like to thank Catherine Giaquinto for producing the excellent figures that illustrate the text. Thank you to Jessica Denning, Ellie Mackie, Mary Mackie and Emmeline Venn for their generous support and providing thoughtful feedback during development.

Many thanks, in advance, to those of you who will engage with all aspects of the GIC (this book, the online learning, the face to face course and the instructor candidacies); no doubt you will have lots of constructive criticism to offer.

Finally we would like to dedicate this book to Mel Humphries who educated alongside us, and inspired so many instructors during a long career as a pioneer educator. Sadly Mel passed away while the book was in its editorial stage, but her voice can still be found within these pages.

CHAPTER 1

Learning

Introduction

By reading this book, you may have already made a decision to reflect on how you teach and learn. You may be thinking about experiences you have had, positive and negative, and want the opportunity to understand why sometimes education is great, and sometimes it really is not. Or perhaps you have been told that you have to read this text and feel just a bit resentful about that. Whatever your motivations this is a chance to explore some of the issues that underpin our responses to education, whether we are teaching, learning or engaged in a bit of both.

Theories of learning have historically been based on observations of the way people learn, and for academics they help to bring some understanding to learning behaviours. The educators who write the curriculums and course materials for life support courses have applied some of these theories to ensure that learning is optimised for our target learners.

In this chapter, we will give a broad overview of relevant learning theories. We will then look in the rest of the book at how we can apply these principles when we are facilitating others.

Pocket Guide to Teaching for Clinical Instructors, Fourth Edition.
Edited by Kate Denning, Kevin Mackie and Alan Charters, Andrew Lockey.
© 2025 John Wiley & Sons Ltd. Published 2025 by John Wiley & Sons Ltd.

First, however, we will consider a number of evidence-based strategies that can be used to make us better learners, so that we can consciously and mindfully use this knowledge when we are teaching.

Learning outcomes

This chapter will enable you to:
- Identify how our brains hold and retrieve information
- Employ effective learning strategies
- Compare and contrast teacher-centred and learner-centred approaches to education
- Consider some of the educational theories that underpin life support courses

---

How we learn

Working memory

It is generally agreed that we have a long-term memory and a working memory (short-term memory). Long-term memory has a limitless storage system. You might, for example, have stored your childhood car registration in your long-term memory and be able to recall it years later. In contrast, working memory is thought to only last around 30 seconds. An example is remembering a phone number for long enough to type it into your phone. Unless this specific piece of information is attended to multiple times it will not pass into long-term memory and will be forgotten.

The role of our working memory is not only to hold pieces of information for a short period but also to *process* that information (i.e. do something with it).

All new memories have to pass through working memory in order to make it into long-term memory. Working memory has a limit and is easily overloaded. Most of us, without any specific brain training, are able to hold in our working memory a surprisingly small number of discrete pieces of information. This has implications for our capacities as learners. If we are presented with too much new information, we cannot process it all. Imagine needing to check the oil level in a car. For somebody who already knows where the dipstick is located and what it looks like, the new information is just the process of checking how far up the oil level reaches. However, for the person who does not know where the dipstick is located, what it looks like, how to open the bonnet of their car, etc., there is a lot more new information to take on and this second person has significantly less working space available to use for processing. It seems inevitable that in this instance they are less likely to retain all of the steps, and therefore to successfully check the oil level, without considerable guidance and input.

Schema

Fortunately, we have ways of managing the limits of our working memory. Our brains are good at finding and forming patterns or structures that help us group pieces of information and understand how complex processes work. This is described as 'chunking'; creating groups or sets of familiar concepts to help retrieve more information, more quickly. We instinctively organise our knowledge, and, as we engage in new learning and take in new information, we connect it to pre-existing knowledge, beliefs or experiences.

Example

If asked to remember a random number such as 48792361 you might struggle. If asked to remember 24681357 it is likely that your brain will 'chunk' this information into 2468 and 1357 so that you are only having to remember two discrete pieces rather than eight separate ones. In order to chunk this information, you will probably have drawn on pre-existing knowledge about number sequencing, odd and even numbers or your 2 times table.

Experts typically have a host of these short cuts which save them expending valuable working memory on too many discrete 'pieces' of information. A professional tennis player does not have to think through all the details of each return shot that they make, they make rapid decisions based on a number of previously experienced episodes. The novice watching them might be overawed by their processing capacity, as they seem able to assess more information with greater speed than a beginner. Essentially, we use existing experience to make sense of new information, and the more experiences we have, the more short cuts we have to draw on. This is a particularly useful concept when trying to make ourselves increasingly adept as learners. It helps if we take as many opportunities as possible to link new learning with knowledge we already have. Equally it helps if teachers or facilitators provide spaces for the learners to make connections that are personal to them.

You may have observed expert team leaders at a cardiac arrest, and noticed their capacity to make quick decisions, rapidly evaluating information through chunking. Their use of schema is essential and efficient, and, through providing structure and frameworks, allows experts to achieve far more than they would if they always had to re-remember and re-process each of the separate elements of any action or knowledge. The problem with this method of information retrieval is that it can lead us to employ stereotypes or make assumptions without always considering the bigger picture. This is referred to as 'cognitive bias' and it is because of concerns about the negative effects of cognitive biases that we need to use the rest of our team to help check our actions and prevent ourselves from making mistakes based on erroneous assumptions. We explore more about cognitive biases, team working and team leadership in the non-technical skills chapter of this book (Chapter 12).

Retrieval practice

The transition from working memory to long-term memory can be arduous but rewarding. For most of us, it is not quite as simple as attending to a piece of information once and then it being miraculously stored in our long-term memory. The information has to be actively retrieved and attended to multiple times in order for it to be fully embedded in long-term memory. This process is referred to as retrieval practice. If you have ever used flashcards to help study for an exam with a question on one side and the answer on the back, you have done retrieval practice. The more this is done the stronger the neural pathways become, and the easier that piece of information is to retrieve.

Sadly, for good learning to occur, anything that feels efficient is likely to be the opposite. Take as an example a habit you may or may not have of reading through a text book in preparation for an exam and highlighting the important bits of information. You might even find that you are highlighting the same bits you identified last time you read it. The act of highlighting is such a low-level activity that very little is required of you in terms of active investment. The chances are that this, like taking photographs of a lecturer's slides, might make you feel good, but will not guarantee that you have learned much. What is far more beneficial in terms of long-term learning is to do any of the following:

- Challenge yourself to write the concepts in your own words, or to draw a concept map
- Make a list of the key facts
- Explain them to a friend or teach a less experienced colleague

These strategies will all take much longer than using a highlighter pen but will avoid what Brown et al. (2014) call 'the illusion of knowing'. Reading something that we have read before feels familiar, we recognise some of it and therefore *feel* like we know it.

Retrieval practice is such a useful tool for us to use because it shifts information into our long-term memory: the more often we retrieve it, the better we learn it; the more connections we make with other pieces of information, the stronger the connections become.

Retrieval practice is also useful as it highlights gaps in our knowledge. If we test ourselves, and do not come up with the right answers, we have clear evidence that we do not know the answer. Unfortunately, as Kruger and Dunning (1999) explain, we are rather bad at judging our own abilities, particularly non-technical skills, and we tend to overinflate our abilities. This is also discussed in more detail in Chapter 12.

Retrieval practice can be done at four different levels of increasing difficulty (Figure 1.1).

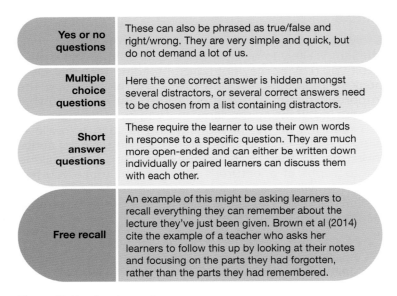

Yes or no questions	These can also be phrased as true/false and right/wrong. They are very simple and quick, but do not demand a lot of us.
Multiple choice questions	Here the one correct answer is hidden amongst several distractors, or several correct answers need to be chosen from a list containing distractors.
Short answer questions	These require the learner to use their own words in response to a specific question. They are much more open-ended and can either be written down individually or paired learners can discuss them with each other.
Free recall	An example of this might be asking learners to recall everything they can remember about the lecture they've just been given. Brown et al (2014) cite the example of a teacher who asks her learners to follow this up by looking at their notes and focusing on the parts they had forgotten, rather than the parts they had remembered.

Figure 1.1 Retrieval practice

Spaced practice

Research has repeatedly shown that for retrieval practice to reap maximum benefits, it is best when it is spaced out over time (see, for example, Bahrick and Hall, 2005). This is the opposite of cramming for an exam, which can be a reasonable strategy if the learner's only goal is to pass the exam the following day. If, however, they need to actually use the knowledge in a variety of contexts, spacing out the practice will ensure they have learnt it more thoroughly. As we will explore throughout this book, contextualising new knowledge and skills in a variety of settings is important for us, both as learners and facilitators.

Spaced practice is a challenge in the design of short courses as, in order for the learning to be most effective, it needs to be revisited on a number of occasions. However, there are still benefits from asking learners to retrieve information that they processed a few hours before, on the previous day or when they were reading the manual. The online resources attached to provider courses deliberately incorporate retrieval practice at the four levels described and spaced practice to maximise learning.

Interleaving

Interleaving, or mixing up what you are learning, is more effective than studying the same subject or topic repeatedly. Kornell and Bjork (2008) illustrated this by asking students to learn to recognise two different artists. Half the group were exposed to paintings by artist A and then paintings by artist B. The other half were shown paintings from both artists in a random pattern. As you would imagine, the latter group were initially more confused and had to work harder to remember which artist had painted which picture. The test came when they were given paintings they had not seen and were asked to identify which artist had done them. Those in the second group were better at identifying the artist correctly, because they had been forced to discriminate between the two throughout the learning phase.

Perhaps the most interesting element of this research is the fact that the students thought that they learnt better when the artists were *not* mixed up... even when they were given the results of the test. This is because 'massed practice' (doing the same thing over and over) is *easier* than interleaving and the 'illusion of knowing' creeps in. Moving onto something new before you have fully grasped the first subject feels frustrating and difficult, but that is precisely when the learning is happening.

Both interleaving and spaced practice work because when we learn something we start to forget it shortly afterwards. Returning to it halts the forgetting, we have to re-learn, but not from quite such a low point as when we started. Each time we re-visit the skill or knowledge we have a small advantage from having already studied or practised it.

Deliberate practice

Deliberate practice has been widely written about, especially in the fields of elite sports, music and chess (Ericsson et al. 1993). In order to become truly accomplished, many hours of practice are required. This is not mindless repetition, or rote learning of the skill, it is a purposeful and thoughtful process of repeating with attention to detail at all phases. Take defibrillation as an example. Here there is a standard 'safe' procedure – check rhythm, restart chest compressions, charge defibrillator, shout 'stand clear', press the shock button. We could easily create assessment criteria that allow candidates to 'pass' or 'fail' based on the process above. What happens, then, when the candidate goes to their first cardiac arrest and the buttons on the defibrillator are in different positions and nobody stands clear when they command it? Deliberate practice would break each component down and allow us to ask ourselves 'what if?' so that our learned behaviour is not just an automatic repetition of a skill that was learned by rote, but builds in contingencies and problem-solving.

Deliberate practice can be incorporated into life support courses in a variety of ways. This might be in the manner that we run sessions or how we manage candidates' practice of certain key skills.

Deliberate practice has a number of elements that need to be present in order for it to be effective (Figure 1.2):

- **Motivation:** You have to be motivated to improve or try something new. You must want to stretch yourself.
- **Focus:** The practice must be focused and thoughtful. This requires working hard.
- **Feedback:** Immediate feedback, whether from internal or external sources, allows you to refine and adapt. If you are open to feedback, you will probably find it much more effective.
- **Repetition:** The more times you do something in different contexts, the better you will become. Spacing out the practice and doing it in different contexts can make you a more mindful practitioner.

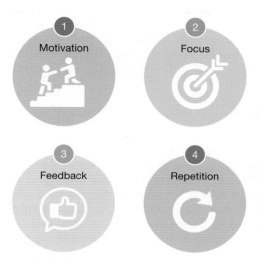

Figure 1.2 Deliberate practice

On life support courses we can offer candidates the opportunity for 'rapid cycle deliberate practice' (RCDP). RCDP is a technique that involves learners performing a simulation or skill, receiving targeted, personalised feedback immediately afterwards and having opportunities to practise the new approach straight away with further feedback being incorporated. In contrast to traditional post-simulation feedback, these feedback sessions are typically more frequent and can be more succinct (de Castro et al., 2022). This offers an opportunity for candidates to be shown how to build up their knowledge and skills into increasingly complex chunks (as was described earlier), builds their expertise and frees up working memory. It also offers the opportunity for candidates who already possess some skills to be coached to a higher level. This is the advantage that deliberate practice offers – feedback can be targeted rather than generic. The feedback should be entirely dependent on the specific needs and current level of expertise of the individual learner, sometimes referred to as 'desirable difficulty'.

Spaced practice and interleaving provide specific ways of introducing desirable difficulties. They introduce impediments into the learning process which make us have to put in more effort, which, in turn, strengthens our learning.

Elaboration

If it is possible to make connections between the current learning experience and prior learning (for example from the online learning, the provider course manual or your own lived experience) then you are engaging in a process described as 'elaboration'. This means that you are really making sense of material that you have learned. The more often you make connections to, or explain a concept, the better you will both understand it and remember it.

It is important, for example, that candidates have the opportunity to make sense of simulated experiences when engaged in post-simulation debrief. If you have ever been frustrated by instructors telling you what you have learnt, or giving their own examples, this is because you have been deprived of the opportunity to build your own, unique understanding. In order to be an effective learner, it is worthwhile taking every available opportunity to make these connections and often the best way of doing this is by talking. Elaboration may also involve creating your own 'story', a concept we explore in more detail below.

Peer teaching

Verbalising plays a key role in the *process* of understanding and, therefore, learning. Explaining a new concept to a fellow learner requires us to make sense of it in our own words. This also allows us to elaborate and create our own narratives and experience. Provider courses offer ample opportunities for peer teaching where instructors are secure enough, and trust the learners enough, to allow learning to happen outside their close supervision.

Stories and concrete examples

Attaching stories to concepts helps us understand them better. These real world examples are often built into books and we have put quite a few in here in the form of examples and case studies. Abstract concepts can be difficult to process unless they are made 'real'. Attaching your own stories to your experiences further enhances your learning and understanding. If, for example, you are trying to understand some of the theoretical concepts in the next section, have a go at drawing on your own experience to come up with examples. This will take a little more time than simply reading the text, but it will help you understand and have a reason for remembering. Incidentally, this will also be a form of elaborating as you make connections between new and old learning.

It is helpful for candidates to have opportunities to bring their own stories to workshops and discussions since this enhances their learning. A simple question such as, *'Has anyone had experience of managing acute asthma?'* will turn out to be a deceptively simple way of securing the learning.

Theories of learning

The next section of this chapter briefly looks at some of the educational theories that have driven the development of life support courses. The strategies already described – retrieving, spacing, verbalising, elaborating, interleaving and story-telling – will be useful for you to employ as you engage with the theories of learning and their application in later chapters.

The scientific study of teaching and learning has been the topic of scholarly research for over 2000 years. A working knowledge of some resulting theories helps us as instructors to understand our own pedagogy. It can help explain why and when certain approaches may be more (or less) effective, thus enabling teaching to be tailored accordingly.

Our favourite teachers were often those who made learning enjoyable and who seemed to speak to us personally. They may have made this look easy, but they probably had substantial knowledge of teaching and learning theories and many years of experience. This section aims to outline some of that educational theory, exploring why and how it underpins our approach to teaching.

As we try to make sense of how we learn and look at some theories of education, it might be helpful to consider seven essentials of teaching and learning:

- Encourage contact between candidates and faculty
- Develop reciprocity and cooperation among candidates
- Encourage active learning (engaging candidates with the course material through discussions, problem-solving, case studies, role play and simulation)
- Give prompt feedback
- Emphasise time on task by keeping as many learners actively engaged as possible
- Communicate high expectations
- Respect diverse talents and ways of learning

(Adapted from Chickering and Gamson, 1987)

Traditional approaches to teaching

A traditional approach to teaching might be described as one in which learners are perceived as 'empty vessels ready to be filled with knowledge'. This is sometimes referred to as a 'didactic' approach, where the teacher tells the learners what they need to know, turning them into passive rather than active participants (Lockey et al., 2021). The lecture is a modality that lends itself to a didactic approach, but as we shall explore in Chapter 10 it does not necessarily have to be.

Objectives and outcomes

The main criticism of a didactic approach is that it is teacher-centred, a 'one size fits all' method with little appreciation of the needs of the learner. In this setting *objectives* are established and the teacher delivers them. By contrast, a learning *outcome* implies that the learners will gain something useful. For example:

Objective: By the end of this session I will have taught you the algorithm

Outcome: By the end of this session you will be able to *remember* the algorithm to help save more lives

Bloom's taxonomy (1956), can be used to provide structure when you are designing learning outcomes as the levels of knowledge are increasingly complex the further you move up the pyramid (Figure 1.3). To illustrate the application of this taxonomy, candidates may be required to demonstrate their *comprehension* of a treatment algorithm before *applying* it and/or *evaluating* its efficacy in different clinical situations.

Bloom's taxonomy is a tool we can use to consider the different cognitive levels that determine the detail and focus of a teaching session. The outcome example above uses the word 'remember'. Consider how replacing 'remember' with 'apply' will influence the content and structure of your session.

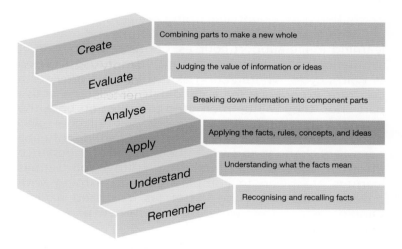

Figure 1.3 Bloom's taxonomy

Andragogy

Andragogy refers to any form of *adult* learning (Knowles, 1984), recognising that most adults have attained wider knowledge and greater experience than children. From a practical standpoint, *andragogy* encompasses a range of approaches that utilise these differences by encouraging *active engagement* in the process and content of learning.

The following is a useful summary of how adults learn:

Adults learn best when:

- They are involved in the planning and evaluation of their learning
- Their own experience (including mistakes) provides the basis for learning activities
- The subject has immediate relevance and impact on their job or personal life
- Learning is problem-centred rather than content-orientated

(Adapted from Knowles, 1984)

Kolb's (1984) experiential learning cycle (Figure 1.4) may be useful in considering how to structure and maximise learning in life support courses. Consider an episode of simulation-based learning that includes the application of Kolb's cycle, where acting as team leader provides a *concrete experience* for a candidate. When the active part ends, they will be prompted to *reflect* on both the activity and their feelings. Through self-reflection and discussion with other candidates, they can identify any necessary changes and relate them to earlier experience (*abstract conceptualisation*). The more opportunities learners are given to compare current learning with previous experience, the better (as discussed earlier). Candidates can then experiment with new or adapted behaviours in future situations.

When teaching adults, consider tailoring your approach to the needs of the particular individual or group involved. For example, during a debrief, if a group of candidates is independently exploring events and having an in-depth clinical discussion, then it may be best for the instructor to remain quiet. Conversely, if salient events have not been raised, the instructor may decide to take a more active role, using language that incorporates good judgement to review the event and encourage further reflection and exploration (Davis & Denning, 2018). This element of debriefing is considered further in Chapter 8.

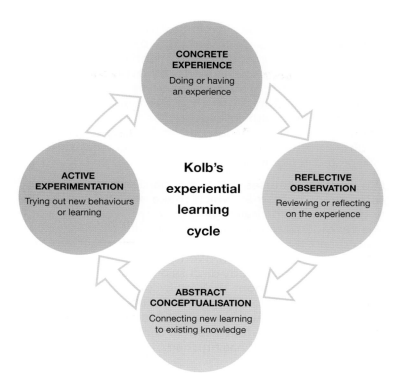

Figure 1.4 Kolb's experiential learning cycle

Heutagogy

Ultimately, today's wide access to learning materials of all kinds means that learners can easily choose their own preferred method of learning, moving beyond being self-directed to becoming self-determined. This has been labelled 'heutagogy'.

Heutagogy is about self-motivated or self-determined learning, the importance of knowing *how* to learn, and how to do it effectively. Recently another strand has arisen: thanks to growing interest in the use of technology, candidates can now choose what, when, where and how they use a variety of resources. However, some candidates appear to find this greater degree of autonomy and flexibility disorientating. They may be either unfamiliar with the new methods or accustomed to approaches used in schools (Chen et al., 2021).

A heutagogical approach has critical thinking and reflection at its heart. Learners are empowered to be analytical about their learning needs and to have a high degree of control over their own learning. This kind of ethos prepares students for the complexities of the ever-changing workplace. It need not be a solo activity, since a key element is collaborating and testing ideas with colleagues, particularly in workshops where learners are encouraged to bring their own case studies, or in simulation where non-technical skills are interpreted in highly personal ways.

Life support courses have standardised learning and assessment outcomes which make aspects of a heutagogical approach challenging. However, we *can* encourage candidates to engage in beneficial activities such as spaced practice, interleaving, retrieval practice, peer teaching and elaboration. We can provide space within workshops for case study discussions that encourage the learners to think about their own contexts so that each learner can work out what they can apply from our sessions. Our courses also direct learners to additional resources and encourage them to continue learning even after the course itself has finished.

Optimising learning

Motivation (sense of purpose)

Motivation is the 'driving force' through which people strive to achieve personal goals, uphold a value or fulfil a need (Ryan & Deci, 2020). This driving force can be *intrinsic* or *extrinsic*. *Intrinsically* motivated candidates attend a course because they actively wish to learn, while *extrinsically* motivated people have usually been told by someone else that they are obliged to attend. Various motivating factors may affect a candidate's attitude and desire/ability to learn; instructors need to consider this when getting to know their candidates. In reality, most people who attend courses probably have a mixture of extrinsic and intrinsic motivators.

Whatever motivation is driving candidates, it is up to instructors to enhance the *desire* to learn, by using interesting and interactive teaching methods and clearly illustrating the clinical benefits of the lessons learned. Also, a genuinely enthusiastic facilitator can be 'infectious', which aids motivation.

Race (2020) places motivation (the 'want' or 'need' to learn) at the centre of efficient learning (Figure 1.5). He argues that candidates learn by doing, and by receiving feedback to help them make sense of what they learn. Learning is deepened by good facilitation, peer teaching (verbalising) and assessment (retrieval practice), all of which are factors in life support courses.

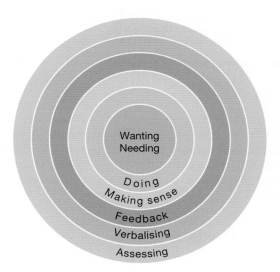

Figure 1.5 Race's ripples model of learning

Sense of security

In order for learning to be maximised, candidates need to feel safe; both physically and psychologically. Maslow's hierarchy of needs (1971) determines that certain fundamental needs must be met to enable candidates to progress (Figure 1.6). With that in mind, life support courses take care to cater for basic physiological needs such as warmth, food, hydration and regular breaks, and to provide them in a physically safe and secure environment.

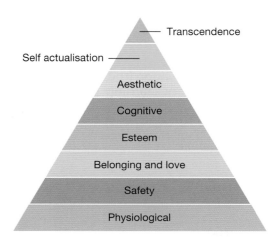

Figure 1.6 Maslow's hierarchy of needs

Psychological and emotional safety are key. Provider courses should be intellectually stimulating and challenging, but candidates also need to feel secure and free to ask questions without threat of criticism or ridicule. The notion of psychological safety is explored more deeply in Chapter 7.

Sense of belonging

In the context of life support courses, a sense of belonging means feeling part of a valued group where new relationships can be formed or existing ones maintained. Creation of this sense of belonging can be challenging, given the timeframes involved and the diverse backgrounds of candidates who may not have met before. However, life support courses are intense, shared experiences that can lead to the formation of strong bonds. To encourage this atmosphere, instructors naturally make use of their emotional intelligence (EI), which means an ability to examine feelings and emotions, to distinguish between them, and to let this information inform actions and decision making (Goleman, 1995).

Mortiboys (2012) regards EI as the third, often unrecognised, component of teaching (the first two being expertise in and knowledge of the subject), and says that its use can result in candidates becoming more motivated, confident, resilient and willing to collaborate. In striving to understand emotions, in both themselves and others, it is helpful for instructors to note how they display their own emotions, in verbal and non-verbal ways. This then also makes it easier to be perceptive to candidates' emotional cues and respond to them appropriately. An example is being able to 'read the room' during a session and then adjust to the ebb and flow of interaction accordingly.

Sense of significance

A sense of significance is achieved when everyone in the group is accorded equal value and status, along with recognition of aspects such as gender equality, diversity, inclusivity and cultural competence. Addressing people correctly conveys that they are valued. Something as apparently simple as using a person's name can be incredibly powerful, creating a sense of belonging and inclusivity. Accurate pronunciation is vital – ask the person how to pronounce their name rather than avoiding or mispronouncing it, and be accepting of correction. This courtesy shows respect and also acknowledges the individuality, identity, race and ethnicity implicit in a name (Bryan, 2021). Of equal importance is the correct use of preferred pronouns during interactions.

Reasonable adjustment

Course design, development and delivery should ensure equality of access and opportunity wherever possible, but in some cases 'reasonable adjustments' may be called for.

With candidates who have dyslexia (for example), there are standard regulations that allow them extra time for written exams. Course directors are a useful resource if you are unsure about what is meant by reasonable adjustments.

Case study

A course centre was approached by a potential candidate who was profoundly deaf. With the agreement of the course director, the candidate arranged to have BSL interpreters available in support. Further discussions were held about ways to ensure the candidate's learning was not compromised by missing peripheral aspects, and that the rest of the group were not compromised by insufficient focus on their needs.

Most governing or awarding bodies offer guidance on making reasonable adjustments, but these are not exhaustive. If the course director is unsure what reasonable adjustments can be made, guidance is usually available when it is sought.

Understanding of these factors and the theories of learning in the wider context will enhance our role as instructors.

Summary and learning

Our brains assimilate and retrieve information in a number of ways.

Having an awareness of how we learn will make us better instructors.

Active engagement in learning is essential for adult learners.

Instructors are pivotal in facilitating responsive learning which reflects the individual needs of the candidates.

In order to optimise learning, instructors are encouraged to consider environmental, social, cultural and interpersonal factors.

CHAPTER 2

Inclusive teaching

Introduction

Take a moment to look around you, at work and at home; you are surrounded by people from diverse backgrounds, who bring with them different perspectives, abilities, talents and contributions. This richness in our communities is often underrepresented, undervalued and underutilised in education and healthcare. In education, research has shown that there are positive consequences to having a learner group that is diverse in terms of culture, neurotype and gender. Cognitive skills and critical thinking are improved because of the more robust interrogation of opinions and perspectives that occurs; in addition, problem-solving skills are enhanced and this leads to improved citizenship. McKinsey and Company (2020) have shown that diverse companies are more likely to financially outperform their peers by up to 28%. Therefore, embracing diversity and making our teaching more inclusive makes sense both for the individual and for the collective.

Pocket Guide to Teaching for Clinical Instructors, Fourth Edition.
Edited by Kate Denning, Kevin Mackie and Alan Charters, Andrew Lockey.
© 2025 John Wiley & Sons Ltd. Published 2025 by John Wiley & Sons Ltd.

> ## Learning outcomes
>
> This chapter will enable you to:
>
> - Describe the considerations you need to make to ensure inclusivity when facilitating
> - Foster an inclusive teaching environment

Inclusive learning

The concept of inclusive learning and teaching has been promoted by various scholars and educational researchers over the years, and its roots can be traced back to the civil rights movement and disability rights advocacy. It has emerged from a long history of advocacy for social justice and equal access to education for all learners.

In healthcare and education, embracing, respecting and valuing diversity is not just a moral imperative but a legal one. In the UK, the Equality Act 2010 clearly states the public sector responsibilities to actively eliminate discrimination and advance equality of opportunity. This duty should be reflected in our approach to learning and teaching through inclusive teaching, wherever in the world we are.

Teaching inclusively

Teaching inclusively means working to ensure that all learners, regardless of their backgrounds or abilities, feel valued and have equal access to educational opportunities.

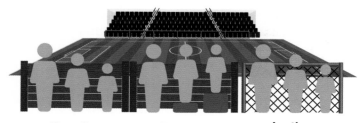

Equality:
everyone is given
the same support

Equity:
everyone gets the
specific support that
they need to thrive

Justice:
the cause of inequality
has been removed

Figure 2.1 Equality, equity and justice

It involves understanding, respecting and responding to the diverse needs of all learners. This may include providing differentiated instruction, creating a safe learning environment and developing accommodations and modifications to support successful learning.

Equality (treating everyone the same) is not the same as equity (providing appropriate and differentiated support) as Figure 2.1 illustrates.

Inclusive learning and teaching recognises that all learners are entitled to an experience that respects diversity, removes barriers, enables participation and anticipates and considers a variety of learning needs and preferences.

UNESCO (2016) outlines a number of factors that should be present for an organisation to be inclusive. They are adapted here as aspirational indicators for an inclusive educational experience (Figure 2.2).

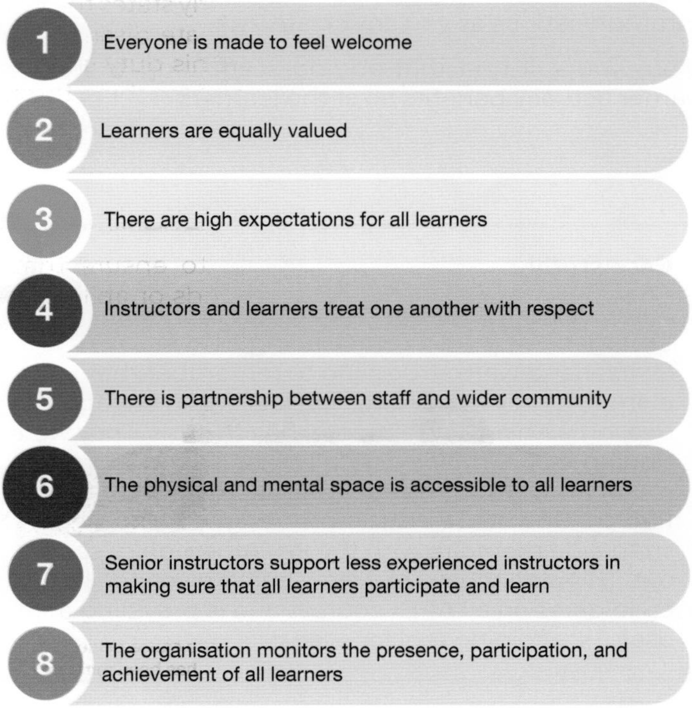

1. Everyone is made to feel welcome

2. Learners are equally valued

3. There are high expectations for all learners

4. Instructors and learners treat one another with respect

5. There is partnership between staff and wider community

6. The physical and mental space is accessible to all learners

7. Senior instructors support less experienced instructors in making sure that all learners participate and learn

8. The organisation monitors the presence, participation, and achievement of all learners

Figure 2.2 Inclusive educational experience

Teaching and learning on all provider courses should reflect these indicators across all aspects of the curriculum.

Differentiated teaching

Given the diversity of your learners, it is up to you as the facilitator to adapt your approach to attempt to meet the needs of all learners. This can be done in several ways.

Reasonable adjustments can be made by providing necessary resources and accommodations to ensure that learners can access the course programme and participate fully in learning activities. This is possible before the course if the question has been asked prior to the learners attending. Asking individuals what accommodations they would like or need is the most important first step; this will help us avoid making assumptions. There could be a wealth of reasons why someone is not responding to your communications as you anticipate.

Often you will find that adding scaffolding to help one learner actually benefits all of the learners.

Case study

Some of the learners on the Acute Psychiatric Emergencies (APEx) course being held in Switzerland were struggling to remember the elements they needed to consider when engaged in dealing with an acute mental health crisis. They were finding it particularly difficult because the source materials were in English awaiting translation to French. One of the instructors designed a pocket-sized aide memoire with the key mnemonics spelt out. This aide memoire is now being given to all candidates on all APEx courses and is providing a useful scaffolding tool for everyone.

It is also important to be aware of our own biases, and challenge ourselves to provide feedback and assessment in a non-biased way. Sometimes we lack the knowledge rather than have a bias, but we need to be open to hearing about a range of responses and perspectives, and to educate ourselves about the conditions. As is explored in Chapter 8, this is best done by using objective criteria (*describing* what you saw/heard) and avoiding assumptions or judgements about a learner's ability based on their background or identity. This is a skill worth attention. It is helpful to remind ourselves that all candidates arrive on courses wanting to learn, they are there hoping to succeed.

Example

ADHD is often misunderstood as a condition that means that the individual cannot concentrate, is disruptive and has poor time management skills. It is in fact a neurodevelopmental disorder that presents with a spectrum of symptoms, which are often interpreted as negative personal qualities. Individuals have years of practice of 'masking' and this can occupy a significant portion of their processing power.

Microaggressions

An awareness of the pervasiveness of microaggressions is important for instructors on provider courses in considering the significance of being a healthy role model.

Microaggressions are '*everyday subtle put-downs directed towards a marginalised group which may be verbal or non-verbal and are typically automatic*' (Sue, 2010). What this means in reality is that microaggressions are so automatic and often so culturally acceptable that people do not even realise that what they are saying may be offensive. Fortunately, our awareness of this is increasing all the time, but a 2017 study of medical students showed 54% of respondents had experienced microaggressions relating to sexism, religion, skin colour and ethnicity (Espaillat et al., 2019). Examples of microaggressions that you may have heard, seen or experienced might be:

- Assuming a female physician is a nurse
- Telling someone they do not look gay
- Telling a person with mental health issues that they cannot be depressed because they are smiling
- Assuming a person who is neurodivergent is either a savant or unable to communicate
- Assuming someone's gender preference from the way they dress

Safe learning spaces

Learners need to feel safe enough to express themselves, take risks and share their knowledge skills and attitudes (Holley and Steiner, 2005). This is described in some detail in Chapter 7. Learners identify a safe space as primarily psychological and emotional rather than physical, although this can also be a component of life support courses.

Providing a safe space does not mean removing the element of challenge for learners. In order for growth and development to happen, there needs to be a balance between challenge and support, but in this context it takes place within a setting in which instructors are respectful, non-biased and approachable. Instructors can and should use their judgement, but need to do this without being judgemental and there is an important difference.

Instructors on life support courses are encouraged to hold all learners on the course in high regard working on the assumption that they are trying to do their best. Where this respectful stance is genuinely held, candidates feel free to treat errors as learning opportunities, rather than mistakes deserving of punishment and shame. This requires the instructor to be mindful of their own unconscious biases and how they may present to a learner. It is difficult to unearth our own unconscious biases and the best ways of doing this are to seek feedback and work with others who have very different life experiences and values. To improve as an instructor, consider deliberately seeking out disconfirming viewpoints and evidence to broaden out how effective you are.

How to create a safe space

To create a space that feels sufficiently safe for all learners, use inclusive language that respects all gender identities, races, religions and cultures. Avoid using language that can be perceived as offensive or exclusionary. For example, avoid using the word 'neurodiversity' to describe learning differences in a group, use neurotype as it is a more inclusive term.

You can build in opportunities for collaborative learning by incorporating group work, peer feedback and teamwork. Encouraging learners to work together in a supportive and inclusive environment encourages them to learn from each other and share their ideas. This can be a real strength of simulation teaching sessions.

Designers of life support courses work hard to incorporate a variety of perspectives, cultures and experiences into their curricula. As an instructor, try to make sure that examples you give come from a variety of cultures and ethnicities and represent a range of abilities. For example, a case study discussion about a seriously ill child who also has complex needs can add to the group's learning because of the additional factors that need to be considered when caring for the child. This would be a good opportunity to model inclusivity by asking the parent and child what they would need.

Accommodations and modifications

The UK Equality Act 2010 makes direct and indirect discrimination on the grounds of protected characteristics unlawful. Therefore, instructors in the UK have a legal obligation to not only be non-discriminatory but to make reasonable adjustments so that no learner is disadvantaged. This law does not apply outside the UK, but the protected characteristics listed are still pertinent in other jurisdictions.

Protected characteristics

- Age
- Disability
- Gender reassignment
- Marriage and civil partnership
- Pregnancy and maternity
- Race
- Religion or belief
- Sex and sexual orientation

Accommodating differing learner needs

If a learner has specific learning or physical needs, then wherever possible course centres and instructors should consider what reasonable adjustments may be made to accommodate those learners. Examples of this are: allowing extra time or building in breaks for examinations; and providing assisted technologies and e-reader compatible materials.

Learners from a range of cultural backgrounds may have differing approaches to learning and may need specific types of support. Some candidates prefer a gentle, roundabout approach to feedback with great care being taken of their sensitivities, others are confused by an approach that does not make it extremely clear what precisely needs changing. This is a challenging tightrope for instructors to walk and means that on occasions you will not get it right. Your best response to these situations in the moment is to be led by the learner, and afterwards to reflect on and identify the moment when things went wrong, i.e. at what point did your approach stop working. This then makes it easier to identify what your alternatives were at that point. We all make mistakes when facilitating and the best that our learners would expect of us is to try and learn from that.

Neurodivergent learners

Neurodiversity is defined as the range of differences in individual brain function and behavioural traits regarded as part of normal variation in humans; it is not pathological but part of the intrinsic diversity in humans. Whilst neurodivergent learners may have specific needs, adopting an inclusive approach is better for all learners. Here are some ways to accommodate neurodivergent learners in your teaching:

- First and foremost, ask the learner what they need in order to succeed. Accommodations should be built around, not imposed upon, the learner
- It is important to provide multiple modes of instruction. Life support courses deliberately use a variety of visual aids, hands-on activities, group discussions and audio recordings, in order to more inclusive
- Provide extra time to process information or complete assignments so that everyone can work at their own pace and reduce stress
- Minimise distractions in the classroom, which will help anyone who is sensitive to sensory stimuli focus on the session
- Allow those with sound sensitivities to use noise-reducing earplugs; this will help minimise sensory input
- Assistive technology, such as text-to-speech software or voice recognition software, can help some learners access and process information more easily
- Consider a flexible approach to assignments and assessments. Providing options for how to demonstrate learning can help everyone showcase their strengths and reduce anxiety
- Some people may have specific triggers that can lead to anxiety or stress. Being aware of these and providing adjustments, such as a quiet space or a designated safe person to talk to, can help them feel supported and reduce stress. The role of the mentor is important here in understanding what specific learning differences may need to be accommodated
- Use concise and unambiguous communication

Some of this may present problems for instructors asking themselves, *'How far is it okay for me to make accommodations?'* This should not be a decision that you have to make on your own, as instructors on life support courses almost always work in pairs. Where a faculty has prior information, and this is usually the case, then they can discuss with each other how they are going to adapt as a team to teaching the group. If nobody has the appropriate knowledge about specific conditions, then it is important to seek it out. If the need to alter a session emerges unexpectedly then make sure that this is shared with other instructors and everyone is kept informed.

Summary and learning

There are some relatively easy adjustments that we can make to our teaching to make it more inclusive.

Fundamentally it helps to find out more about individual learners' needs and make sure that everyone feels respected and valued.

Be prepared to make adaptations to suit the context of the individual learner, it may also result in improvements for all of the learners.

CHAPTER 3

Facilitating learning

Introduction

This chapter sets out the practical principles of facilitating learning as used throughout the book. The framework of 'Prepare, Open, Facilitate and Close' can be used in most sessions, including lectures, workshops, skill stations and simulations.

Facilitating learning is often referred to simply as 'teaching' but the concept of facilitation of learning implies a more learner-centred approach. Despite this, the terms 'facilitation' and 'teaching' are often used synonymously. Merriam and Brockett (2007) say that adult learning is *'a practice in which adults engage in systematic and sustained self-educating activities in order to gain new forms of knowledge, skills, attitudes, or values'*. However, there is still a need for education that follows a specific curriculum with associated learning outcomes which may or may not be assessed. Spencer (2006) defines this as 'formal learning': *'Structured learning that typically takes place in an education or training institution, usually with a set curriculum and [that] carries credentials'*. This reflects the teaching and learning for most life support courses

Pocket Guide to Teaching for Clinical Instructors, Fourth Edition.
Edited by Kate Denning, Kevin Mackie and Alan Charters, Andrew Lockey.
© 2025 John Wiley & Sons Ltd. Published 2025 by John Wiley & Sons Ltd.

and, in order to deliver an effective session, some care and attention must be taken to ensure that the structure of your session maximises the opportunities for learning.

Learning outcomes

This chapter will enable you to:

- Formulate and structure a teaching session using the format of:
  - Prepare
  - Open
  - Facilitate
  - Close

A teaching structure

In the previous editions of this book, we talked about 'Environment, Set, Dialogue and Closure' as the phases of a teaching session. This led to some confusion as 'Set' was misunderstood by instructors and candidates to mean 'setting up', which is clearly more about the environment than about starting the session. In this edition, we hope that 'Prepare, Open, Facilitate and Close' offer a less ambiguous and more active approach to structuring a session.

The principles remain very similar – a structured approach helps both teachers and learners to navigate the session with more meaningful outcomes. Let us now consider each phase in more detail.

Prepare

Preparation starts as soon as you are allocated to lead or teach a particular session. Planning and preparedness may include: yourself, the environment, your teaching materials, the learners and any assessment criteria/materials.

Yourself: It may seem obvious, but in order to be an effective teacher, you must know your subject. Take time to remind yourself of the core learning outcomes associated with the session and immerse yourself in the subject matter. As a life support instructor you are expected to know the current guidelines and be able to deliver most of the course's core content. If, as a less experienced teacher, you find this rather intimidating, you may prefer to renegotiate your teaching assignments with the course director. A lesson plan is a useful way to scope your session in advance and will help you plan for most eventualities while taking into account the time constraints of the timetable. Also, take the opportunity to update yourself on any changes in course materials or teaching approaches.

The teaching environment: An integral part of the teaching and learning experience is the environment. You should consider aspects such as heating, lighting, ventilation, acoustics, simulation aids and the arrangement of furniture. These issues all relate to the physiological needs of your candidates.

The physical environment can radically affect how a teaching session is conducted and how it will be received. For example, rows of chairs restrict participation, whereas a circle implies that everyone is expected to contribute. Inadequate heating and lighting can undermine a teaching session which has otherwise been meticulously prepared. Students who cannot hear the instructor or see a demonstration will find it difficult to achieve the learning outcomes.

The teacher must endeavour to make the environment as conducive to learning as possible, but sometimes in a particular setting you may not be able to set an optimum environment. For example, many hospitals and universities have poorly regulated heating with cramped or cluttered training rooms. Be mindful of any confounding factors and do your best to compensate for deficiencies.

Teaching materials: Make sure that you have the equipment you need for the whole session. This may include flip charts, pens, handouts, clinical equipment and manikins. Many establishments have their own technical complexities, which can be especially frustrating if you are using electronic teaching media. In hospitals and universities IT systems are sometimes locked down or encrypted; relying on bringing a presentation on a 'memory stick' may not be appropriate. Find out in advance if there are specific local issues that need to be considered. You should also check that Wi-Fi is available and accessible, especially important with the increasing use of online and hand-held devices. If you are using clinical equipment during a skill or simulation session, it is important to check that everything you need is available and functioning so that you give the learners the best possible experience.

The learners: There is usually a requirement for learners to complete pre-course online learning and, at the least, to have read pre-course information and materials such as the course manual. Course organisers should make sure that learners are clear what preparation is expected of them and give them sufficient time to prepare by sending pre-course information in a timely manner. This is usually at least four weeks before the start of any formal face to face teaching. It is also useful for the candidates to have prior knowledge of the assessment strategies and outcomes that will be used on the course.

Assessment materials: Make sure that you know whether your session is linked to any assessment criteria. Familiarise yourself with the associated materials so that you know what the assessed outcomes of your session are.

Open

This is about creating the psychological conditions within which learning can be maximised. Some of the main components to consider are:

- Atmosphere
- Motivation
- Learning outcomes
- Roles
- Timing

These are established in the first few minutes of any session. It is during this time that the instructor will generate the *atmosphere* and enhance the learners' *motivation* by demonstrating the usefulness of the content for them. Emphasise the significance of the session, how it fits into the programme as a whole and what learners may expect from the session. In this phase, the *learning outcomes* will be stated, outlining the territory to be explored.

Learners also need to understand their *role*, for example: your expectations on their interactions; their part in any 'role play' that might take place; and whether they are being assessed formatively or summatively. You should remind learners to be themselves and give support to their fellow learners, thereby fostering an inclusive and compassionate teaching environment. If there is to be role play from the instructors, the purpose and parameters of this activity must be clearly explained for everyone's benefit.

Ensure that the *timing* and the planned duration of the session is adhered to and is understood by learners. If you have to curtail the session rather abruptly because of time constraints, and the candidates have not been warned that this might happen, they may feel this was due to something they did or did not do.

Facilitate

The main part of the teaching session involves interaction between the learners and teacher, which allows learning outcomes to be achieved. This is the central core of the session and will be by far the longest phase.

There are many ways of 'facilitating' the core elements. Methods differ depending on the teaching modality (lecture, workshop, skill station, simulation, assessment, etc.). Irrespective of the technique used, the instructor must ensure that the content is available to the learner in a clear and logical form, and at a level which can be understood. This aspect is explored more fully in chapters dealing with the different modalities.

Checking whether the ideas have been understood, and creating opportunities for retrieval practice, usually involves questions and answers in one form or another. It is important to respond appropriately to candidates' questions in ways that promote learning. An example of this might be a question about a particular drug or procedure. The answer should add context and meaning rather than just being a 'give this', 'do that' response.

Good facilitation is a subtle blend of questions (not interrogation) and teaching. Quickly filling in gaps in learners' knowledge to allow them to progress, or getting their colleagues to help solve problems, can be productive approaches.

Life support courses run to fairly tight schedules. Care should be taken to ensure that each candidate has an equal amount of time to achieve required outcomes. An example of this is a simulation teaching session with two scenarios, timetabled for 30 minutes. If you spend 20 minutes on the first scenario, the next candidate will have 50% less time; this is not fair. Time being one of the hardest elements to manage, instructors must always know when their sessions are due to start and finish. Course directors and coordinators often help by giving regular time markers. These are not to be ignored; most time is lost simply by instructors talking too much.

Close

Having facilitated your candidates to achieve the outcomes for the session, a structured closure will allow for: final questions; summary of key points; communication of any assessment decisions; and termination. A session that does not end clearly will probably have an unsatisfactory feel about it and may leave unanswered questions in the students' minds. Some learners and instructors may find the mnemonic 'QRST' a good way of remembering the structure of closure:

- Questions
- Response
- Summary
- Termination

A period for questions from the learners allows any remaining problems to be aired and responded to. Taking questions *before* summarising the session means that the last message the learners receive is a positive one. If we ask for questions *after* summarising, learners may be confused or focused on the answer to a particularly tricky or irrelevant question. It is important to give learners time to formulate questions and not be afraid to wait in silence while they think. Learners may need longer than a couple of seconds; asking for questions and waiting somewhere between 5 and 10 seconds is probably beneficial.

A concise summary revisits the learning outcomes, pulls together the key points of the session and relates them to other parts of the course. If assessment decisions were part of the required outcomes for the session, the candidate's success or failure to meet them must also be clearly communicated. This is particularly important with serial outcomes-based or continuous assessment and this is further explored in Chapter 9. As instructors we should not forget that candidates may reflect on a session and later, in one of the breaks for example, ask about the clinical scenario or their own or their team's performance. Reflection should be encouraged as it is an important facet of learning. Some courses, such as the Generic Instructor Course (GIC), encourage written reflection and most courses have learning support or mentor meetings where there should be time to reflect.

Finally, 'termination' ends the session. This can be achieved in a variety of ways, the most obvious being a direct verbal instruction linked with a break in eye contact and a physical move away from the group. Termination can be achieved quite simply by saying *'Thank you, that ends the session, you are now going to...'*

Summary and learning

A structured approach can be applied to all teaching interventions: Prepare, Open, Facilitate, Close will help to optimise learning outcomes.

CHAPTER 4

Facilitating workshops and small groups

Introduction

Working in groups can be an effective method of learning, particularly for professionals in a multidisciplinary environment. The outcomes of well-organised group activity can be better than those achieved by an individual member working alone. It is also recognised that group activity can be extremely useful in assessing a learner's ability to apply theoretical knowledge to practice. To achieve these goals, this teaching method requires the instructor to be a facilitator of learning rather than a definitive source of knowledge. The challenge, therefore, is to create a setting where candidates benefit from a more learner-centred experience than, say, a lecture, however interactive that might be.

Learning outcomes

This chapter will enable you to:

- Describe how to run an effective workshop or discussion
- Identify approaches to use when facilitating a group to maximise learning
- Explain group dynamics that might occur within a workshop or small group

Facilitating small groups

The key to successful and productive workshops and small groups is that attention is centred on the candidates doing the work, not on the expert talking about their own expertise. A cooking workshop means learners cook things and a writing workshop means students write things. If most of a 'workshop' is people not actually doing anything, it should perhaps be called a class, a lecture, or a mistake. Many experts lack experience in facilitating workshops because they are used to lecturing, when the spotlight is on the speaker; a workshop turns that spotlight onto each of the learners. For this reason, the skills involved in planning and facilitating workshops and discussions are very different. Instead of creating a message for people to listen to, a good workshop gives learners the opportunity to solve problems for themselves, thus increasing their understanding.

Adult learners bring a wealth of personal experience to the classroom and it is important to recognise and build on this: group activities are far better than many other approaches. As in all educational settings, good planning, organisation and facilitation are required. The ideal group size is probably four to ten learners, although with groups of more than six the layers of interaction become more complex, and groups of three or fewer may be difficult to facilitate.

This chapter explores the different approaches to facilitating small groups, providing some ideas for preparation and planning, whilst highlighting the skills required of the facilitator.

Work mode

Some workshops may be based around a problem-solving approach. In those cases, a clinical scenario or case allows learners to apply their own knowledge and explore treatment strategies based on current treatment guidelines. The facilitator must resist the temptation to 'teach' the candidates as it is much more fruitful if candidates are empowered to voice their own thoughts as long as the group is maintained in 'work mode'. Wilfred Bion (1952, 1967) suggests that groups work in two distinct ways, which he called 'basic-assumption mode' and 'work mode'. Basic assumption mode describes the way the group behaves when they are *avoiding* work. There are three distinct ways in which this happens: flight/fight, dependence and pairing. He believed that these modes undermine a group's capacity to achieve its purposes. You may have witnessed flight/fight where learners are not entirely clear what they need to achieve and become distracted and start to work 'off task'. Groups operating in the 'dependency' basic assumption look to the leader (facilitator) to do all the work for them. Leaders often comply with this and inadvertently prevent the group from working independently. 'Pairing' is a somewhat more complex basic assumption, seen occasionally in groups when two members take over and appear to be providing the answers and direction for everyone. Clear outcomes and vigilant facilitation are the key to keeping the group in 'work mode' whilst an awareness of the way the group is behaving may be useful in understanding the dynamics at play.

Most life support courses involve significant amounts of small group work, whether it be skills stations, workshops, table top discussions or simulations. There are also other opportunities when groups form for less structured input, for example, during faculty meetings, mentor meetings and other ad hoc sessions. These may require less overt structure and facilitation, but the content of these small group interactions still needs careful management and consideration of group dynamics.

As with all teaching modalities, attention needs to be paid to four elements: Prepare, Open, Facilitate and Close.

A teaching structure: workshops and small groups

Prepare

Some consideration needs to be applied to the seating position of candidates to allow them to engage with each other, with the facilitator and with any teaching materials or audiovisual aids being used. Productive layouts include a horseshoe or circle, but in both cases it is important to avoid people obscuring each other's view (Figure 4.1). If using a circle layout, leave a small gap to prevent candidates feeling 'trapped'. This gap also allows them to leave the group with minimal disruption if they become distressed, suffer sensory overload or need to take a break.

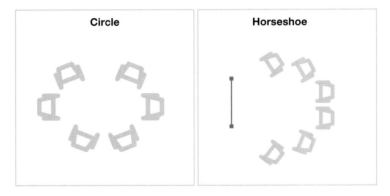

Figure 4.1 Possible layouts for seating in small groups

Common aids used to focus the session include: flip chart, electronic media (computer/laptop/tablet), whiteboard, printed handouts, course materials and clinical resources or props. Instructors should be clear about when they will introduce props or handouts into a session. In some cases, printed algorithms might be used to direct a session towards specific treatments, whilst other sessions might use a handout as a summary of key treatments. If a handout, such as an ECG strip, is to be given to candidates, instructors need to make sure that they have finished speaking before passing it round so that the aid does not turn into a distraction.

Open

In some respects, the beginning might be the most important contribution the instructor will make in establishing successful group work as group norms emerge early in any session (we will return to norms later). We have already stated the importance of concise learning outcomes. Make sure that they are clearly articulated. The phrase *'This session will enable you to...'* will help you to set realistic and achievable outcomes.

It is helpful to include quick introductions, which serve two purposes:

- Gives everyone the opportunity to 'hear their voice' in the group. This allows them to claim 'air time' and gives them permission to speak again
- Allows the facilitator to make some assessment of the group's individual and collective experience and 'mood'

The initial phase of small group work in online settings (Chapter 11) differs from face to face group work in one significant way. It may be the case that some group members do not really feel they are 'present' until they have spoken. The fact that people can be both there and not there, seen and not seen, has potential consequences for the ease and flow of the conversation. By ensuring that everyone has spoken within the first minute, the chances of them feeling anchored within the session increases.

Some thought needs to go into your opening comments and questions, and how you will engage the candidates' interest in the topic. Describing a case, or asking if anyone has a relevant example from their own experience, can be a useful hook for drawing people in. As was described in Chapter 1, most of us respond to personal experience and anecdotes, and these are particularly fruitful when they originate from within the group.

Other elements are more subtle, demanding as much attention to *how* you say something as to *what* you say. It is the facilitator's role to remain alert to patterns of participation (including their own) and to encourage healthy norms, especially at the start of the session.

Norms and ground rules

Norms are different from ground rules, especially those that are announced formally at the beginning of a session. Ground rules represent an aspiration, for example *'We will not talk over each other'*, whereas norms are features of how people collectively behave: they often do talk over each other, with individuals telegraphing the desire to speak by gently interrupting/agreeing with the current talker (see boxes below for examples of ground rules and norms). This does not *necessarily* represent a problem as it increases the energy in the room. Norms are not intrinsically good or bad, they are just the normal behaviour in that group at that time. It is usual for the norms to differ slightly from group to group (Tuckman and Jensen, 1977). The key skill for the facilitator is being vigilant about the norms that emerge from the interaction in the group and if necessary (and possible) attempting to reshape them if they are unhelpful. The challenge is that norms are implicit rather than explicit.

Examples of ground rules	**Examples of norms**
• Everyone will arrive on time for the session	• One person arrives late for all the sessions
• Everyone's voice is equally important	• The facilitator's voice is more important than everyone else's
• Talk-time will be shared out equally among the group	• Some people talk more than others
• Everyone will respect each other	• Everyone clearly respects each other

Facilitate

One of the important features of small group work is the focus on facilitating the group to engage in meaningful dialogue within and amongst themselves. Most life support courses have specific sessions that revolve around clinical cases, table top exercises, pathologies or specific clinical interventions. Having established the parameters of the topic, it is the construct of questions posed by the facilitator that moves a session beyond an interrogation into an interesting and informative discourse.

An awareness of different question styles and types (Figures 4.2 and 4.3), based on Bloom's taxonomy (Chapter 1) will increase the options open to the facilitator.

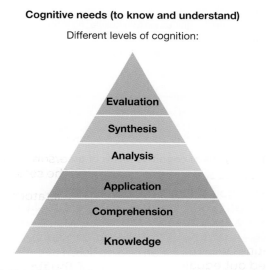

Cognitive needs (to know and understand)

Different levels of cognition:

Evaluation

Synthesis

Analysis

Application

Comprehension

Knowledge

Figure 4.2 Cognitive needs

It will be clear to you that if your opening question is a knowledge-level question, there is not going to be much interaction. For example, '*What is the capital of Norway?*' Equally, if you ask a very high-level question (synthesis or evaluation), it may be beyond all or most of your group. For example, '*What is the meaning of life?*'

Often, then, questions pitched at the level of comprehension, application and analysis are what is required to encourage learners to engage with one another and to help them achieve the learning outcomes of the session.

Analysis
· What are the most significant elements of advanced life support?
· How can we prioritise the management of a challenging resuscitation?
· Compare and contrast the approaches to resuscitation in adults and children.

Application
· Has anyone had any experience of managing a major incident?
· Based on the guidelines for choking, how could we devise an action plan?
· What actions could you take to correct a PaO_2 of 82%?

Comprehension
· How would you describe ventricular fibrillation?
· What do you understand by the term 'delayed cord clamping'?
· What would be an example of a clinical feature of anaphylaxis?

Figure 4.3 Examples of cognitive levels of questions

Instructors should aim to avoid asking too many simple questions with short answers that require little thought. This is not a good use of the small group environment where we should be encouraging candidates to analyse and contextualise their learning, to listen to each other and build an enhanced understanding of the topic. Compare two examples:

Example questions

'What do you think are the treatment options for life-threatening asthma?'

'Given X case, can you prioritise the treatment options and give your rationale for your decisions?'

On the surface both questions are asking about treatment options, but the second demands a much more in-depth group analysis and would form the basis of an absorbing discussion within a workshop.

Asking the group to divide into pairs to discuss a specific issue is a useful strategy for a range of situations because of the importance of verbalising and elaboration already described in Chapter 1 (Figure 4.4).

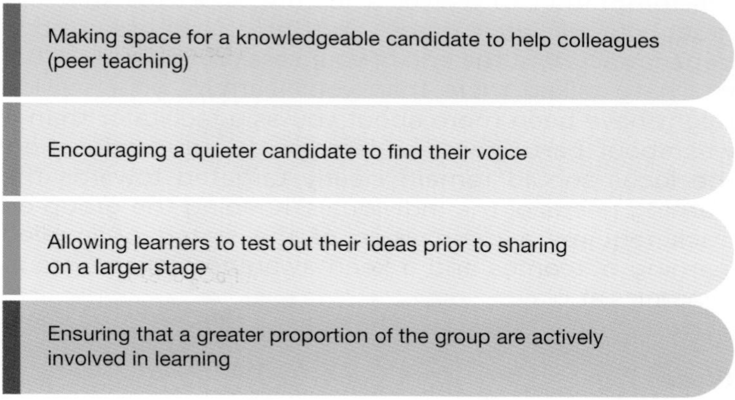

Making space for a knowledgeable candidate to help colleagues (peer teaching)

Encouraging a quieter candidate to find their voice

Allowing learners to test out their ideas prior to sharing on a larger stage

Ensuring that a greater proportion of the group are actively involved in learning

Figure 4.4 Advantages of paired discussions

It is helpful for the instructor leading the session to provide brief summaries of specific elements before refocusing the group on a different aspect of the topic (these are often referred to as 'micro-summaries'). Equally, if the group has been divided and then brought back together, it might be appropriate to ask each subgroup to provide a summary of their work before moving on. In some sessions, where there has been a healthy discussion and some ambiguity remains, it is appropriate to make sure 'concrete' messages are communicated if they will be assessed during the course.

David Kolb, an American social scientist famous for introducing the 'experiential learning cycle' (Chapter 1) talked about the nature of facilitation and related it to the notion of the dinner party host. In Kolb's view, this role was to create an environment, provide food and drink and invite the right combination of guests. The role during dinner was more enabling: ensuring food and drink arrived in a timely manner, gently refereeing, when required, and bringing the evening to a satisfactory conclusion.

This metaphor may help you think through the process of small group management. The key element to keep in mind is that *you* should not be the centre of attention; rather you should be a relatively silent presence, who listens attentively and contributes when necessary in order to redirect, refocus or bring to a conclusion. The most common pitfall for the instructor in small groups is the temptation to deliver a lecture and thus shift the group out of 'work mode' and into basic assumption dependency. If, at the end of your session, you realise that you have talked more than your learners, your session might have been more about you as a facilitator than it was about participants as learners. In adult education, the focus should remain clearly targeted towards the learning needs of the individuals. Keeping the group on track requires a clear vision of the stated or implied learning outcomes and a keen awareness of the group dynamics at play.

Close

When you are closing a workshop or small group session it is useful to clarify any points or answer any questions that may be raised. If there are any unresolved issues, these should be dealt with before summarising and terminating the session. For a summary, you might find it useful to ask the candidates what they have learned from the session rather than just listing the things that you hope you covered. Termination of workshops/small groups is managed in the same way as other sessions.

Group dynamics

Managing groups can be quite complex. An effective session usually requires group members to have done some preparation by pre-reading; the purpose of the workshop or small group session is to check their understanding and clarify any uncertainties through discussion among themselves. After the instructor's initial questions, a subtle use of body language allows the conversation to develop among the candidates, having them speaking to one another, rather than directing everything to you.

With small group work, one of the questions we could consider is: '*What is the nature of the intellectual activity that candidates are engaging in?*'

In lectures, this is relatively straightforward: candidates listen, consider, compare with existing knowledge and either accept or reject the conclusions – usually the former. In small group work, however, it is not simply a matter of rehearsing what has been previously read, it is about exploring understanding and promoting conversation or discussion.

> '*Discussion encourages [learners] to organise their thinking by comparing ideas and interpretations with each other and [helps] to give expression, and hence form, to their understanding of a subject.*'
> (Jacques, 2015)

We engage in conscious and unconscious behaviours and often, but not always, are aware of the effect of our body language, carefully chosen words, intonation and how we listen. Particular attention needs to be paid to these facets to avoid a negative impact on the group. Some helpful strategies include:

- Make frequent sweeps of the group at eye level but do not retain eye contact with a person who is speaking. This makes people speak to the group rather than to you
- Consider your posture: leaning forward is affirming (but may make the facilitator the focus); leaning back may encourage the group to talk to each other
- Avoid validating every contribution as this may stifle contributions and prevent further exploration

The term 'paralinguistics' is used to encompass the non-verbal elements of communication which include: body language, gestures, facial expressions and tone and pitch of voice. When facilitating learning, the paralinguistic features of language are important as they can change the message completely. For candidates whose first language is different from yours, the nuance of pitch and tone may be lost. Clarity and pace of speech may help, as will avoiding slang and jargon or mnemonics that have no meaning in other languages.

Maximising candidate engagement

Many instructors worry about maintaining control: that if the group is encouraged to talk amongst themselves, chaos may reign. This is usually down to expectations or fears about challenging candidate behaviours. We will briefly look at candidates who contribute too much, create distractions or do not speak at all.

Candidates contributing too much

You want people to talk. If, however, someone contributes more than is appropriate, this can prevent the rest of the group from having the opportunity to engage. Often people talk out of enthusiasm, and sometimes they are not aware that they are hindering the contributions of others. There are a number of strategies that you can use once you realise that an individual is dominating:

- Thank them for their contribution and invite others to comment
- Reduce or remove eye contact for a period of time
- Avoid getting into a one-to-one dialogue with them
- Turn away slightly so you are orientated towards another part of the group
- Slightly raise a hand, palm down, or gently touch the person (this is a culturally specific intervention to be used with caution)
- With care it is sometimes possible to use humour

In most situations, candidates just want to engage and learn. The strategies outlined are usually successful, but they do take a bit of time to get right.

Candidates creating distractions

You may encounter distractions such as whispering, answering phone calls, texting, fiddling with equipment, etc. However, be sensitive to the individual needs of learners; some may have specific learning differences or neurodivergent qualities which might be interpreted as distractions.

In order to avoid making assumptions it is always worth checking/asking before judging. If, for example, a candidate is using a mobile phone to take notes, this is legitimate use of electronic media and a simple question to the candidate may resolve what you have perceived as a potential distraction.

When working with a group of adults, an early strategy to address distractions may be to ignore the behaviour which might cease naturally. Additionally, you can try asking a direct question or could build an activity into the session that may refocus the group on the learning outcomes and keep them in 'work mode'.

Candidates who do not contribute

Some candidates may be quite reflective in nature and a lack of verbal contribution should not necessarily be taken as an indication of non-engagement. If a candidate has not contributed to the session and you wish to give them an opportunity to do so, you can encourage them by:

- Giving eye contact
- Turning towards that person
- Offering an open hand (palm up)
- Asking *'Does anyone on this side of the room have any experience?'*
- Saying *'[Name], in your experience, what have you seen happen?'*

If you notice that a previously quiet person looks as if they are about to speak, make sure that you return to them and give them the opportunity to join in.

Although it is important to engage all of the candidates in the group, none of them should be 'forced' to contribute. It is not essential for everyone to make a contribution as long as they are being attentive and have been given the appropriate opportunity to speak.

The exception to this comes when there is an assessed component of the workshop, and then it must be made clear to the candidates what level of participation is required of them in order for you to make an appropriate assessment decision.

The main aims of any small group or workshop are to cover the necessary learning outcomes, encourage group interaction and keep them in 'work mode'.

Summary and learning

Design your session around clear learning outcomes.

Facilitation requires you to: create the right environment, pose the right questions and actively listen.

An awareness of group dynamics will assist you in managing groups.

Keeping the group engaged and focused in 'work mode' may require sensitive interaction from the facilitator.

Micro-summaries and redirection can help keep the group focused on the learning outcomes.

CHAPTER 5

Learning skills

Introduction

Patient safety outcomes are influenced by the quality of technical skills and procedures carried out by healthcare professionals. The extent to which we acquire practical skills is influenced by retention of relevant knowledge, psychomotor performance and the attitude of the learner. Regular practice of the skill maintains and improves performance. Psychomotor learning theory (Simpson, 1972) underpins the approach to skills teaching and assessment outlined in this chapter. Deliberate, repeated practice of a skill helps to ensure that it is embedded in long-term memory.

Life support courses have historically promoted a didactic approach to the teaching of skills using what was described as a 'staged' approach. In this chapter we will explore alternative staged or 'stepwise' approaches that focus more on the learners' needs. Good responsive skills teaching needs to be hands-on, immersive and engaging.

Pocket Guide to Teaching for Clinical Instructors, Fourth Edition.
Edited by Kate Denning, Kevin Mackie and Alan Charters, Andrew Lockey.
© 2025 John Wiley & Sons Ltd. Published 2025 by John Wiley & Sons Ltd.

> ## Learning outcomes
>
> This chapter will enable you to:
>
> - Describe the importance of skills teaching
> - Consider relevant educational theories related to the acquisition of psychomotor skills
> - Choose a strategy for skills teaching that meets the needs of the curriculum and the learner
> - Identify when to correct errors and give feedback in skills development

Attitudes towards learning new skills

Understanding the learner's prior experiences acknowledges how past experiences shape current and future learning events. Simpson refers to this as understanding the learners' 'readiness to act'. Recognising learners' differing attitudes allows us to modify our teaching approach so that it aligns as far as possible with the learner's current level of development. This can be achieved at the beginning of either a skill or simulation teaching session by enquiring about current level of competence in the skill. On life support courses, some of the learners may routinely perform particular skills in their normal working environment, whereas others may not have had the opportunity to do so. Acknowledging each learner's professional background and expertise will improve motivation by tailoring the learning session more closely to their needs.

Stages of psychomotor learning

Psychomotor learning occurs at the crossover between cognitive function and physical movement. Key factors that influence skills acquisition include the amount of practice, the task complexity and feedback. Simpson (1972) suggests learners go through three key stages in learning a skill – 'cognitive', 'associative' and 'automatic' – and that learners imitate instructor behaviours through repeated 'trial and error'.

The cognitive stage

This stage really starts with a comprehension of what the skill is and why it is performed. This is often addressed in pre-course learning or in-course demonstration by faculty members. Some life support courses use instructors embedded within teams to facilitate in situ performance (demonstration) of particular skills.

When it comes to acquiring the skill, large amounts of mental energy may go into getting the motor movements right. Therefore, whilst trying to remember both the sequence of events and the movements required, the learner may appear slow and clumsy. The facilitator can offer support by guiding and correcting them and making use of any cognitive aids that free up the learner's working memory, for example using a printed algorithm. Candidates need encouragement, so at this stage the facilitator's role is instilling confidence, increasing motivation, encouraging participation and emphasising the acquisition of the skill as it develops. Many learners will be familiar with the procedures involved even if they have never done them themselves. Overanalysing the first attempt may be counter-productive and a combination of encouragement and trial and error can be very effective. It is tempting to assume that the cognitive stage is all about instructors telling candidates what they need to do, when it is actually about learners making sense of the skill whilst performing it themselves.

The associative stage

In the associative stage, learners use prior experience to help them improve. Feedback from the teacher should continue to be encouraging whilst learners are developing the ability to provide their own feedback. A useful question at this stage is *'How did that feel?'* which encourages the learner to evaluate their own performance, and the facilitator to offer helpful suggestions. This is where learners can practise and hone their skills and begin to relate them to their own clinical or simulated practice. With skills teaching on life support courses, progress is often 'continuously assessed' and learners may experience the associative stage during independent practice in simulations.

The automatic stage

The automatic stage occurs when the learner undertakes a skill without having to think about it, when it has become embedded into long-term memory and has evolved into unconscious practice. This stage leaves room for further adaptation and refinement, where professionals can start to think about adapting to unforeseen problems. They are now at the height of their practice and will value focused and analytical feedback to make further refinements through the process described in Chapter 1 as 'rapid cycle deliberate practice' (RCDP). They may also begin to help other colleagues/candidates to achieve their goal. As identified earlier, this process of peer teaching is an invaluable part of learning.

The psychomotor domain

The psychomotor domain (Simpson, 1972) includes physical movement, coordination and use of the motor-skill areas of the brain (frontal lobe and cerebellum). On life support courses, development of such skills requires analysis and is measured in terms of speed, precision, distance, procedures or techniques. Thus, psychomotor skills range from manual tasks, such as inserting an i-Gel or doing chest compressions, to more complex tasks such as operating a defibrillator or intraosseous device safely.

Teaching methods

A staged or stepwise approach to teaching psychomotor skills is widely accepted and used in life support courses. A number of models exist, but they share common principles:

- Teach progressively from the simple to the complex
- Teach skills in the order in which they will be used
- Employ continual reinforcement
- Integrate cognitive and psychomotor learning
- Encourage confident employment of the skills
- Repeated analysis improves competence

Staged (stepwise) approach to teaching skills

You may remember from Chapter 1 a description of the limits in processing capacity of working memory, or cognitive load. The facilitator needs to break down complex tasks to make the skill accessible. Importantly, new motor skills need to be practised in short and frequent episodes. Ideally a period of time is left between attempts (spaced practice) and if skills are combined (in the process we have already referred to as interleaving) this also may enhance learning.

Preparatory work:

- Identify the learners' experiences and needs in relation to the skill. Nicholls et al. (2016) suggest special attention is paid to learners who may have developed incorrect practices. They suggest observing the learner's current technique prior to teaching, a method known as 'trial and error, followed by feedback'
- Review all key information linked to competent skill execution (including equipment handling) and related anatomy/physiology

Following this familiarisation, some of which may have occurred prior to face to face teaching, facilitation is initiated by the instructor. The aim is to gradually hand over cognitive and motor elements to the learner, thus supporting their journey to independent practice.

Fitts and Posner (1967) described the stages of skills acquisition. Walker and Peyton (1998) translated this model into a four-stage approach to skills teaching that has been widely used on life support courses (Bullock, 2000). This approach still has some merit, especially for novices. The four stages are:

Stage 1: the instructor demonstrates the skill as usually carried out

Stage 2: the instructor repeats the skill with explanation

Stage 3: the candidate/s provide commentary whilst the instructor performs the skill

Stage 4: the candidates practise under supervision

Modifications to the 'four-stage approach'

Breckwoldt et al. (2023) undertook a systematic review of skills teaching methods and identified that there was no statistically significant difference between Peyton's four-step approach and a number of alternative stepwise strategies. They recommend that a stepwise approach to skills teaching is used for resuscitation training, but that Peyton's four-step approach may not always be the preferred one.

For candidates undertaking a Generic Instructor Course (being assessed on the way they teach skills), a clear framework for such teaching is required.

Demonstration

In life support courses, a demonstration does not always have to be delivered during skills teaching if it has been embedded within a simulation or previewed by the learners on the e-learning platform. It is worth asking your candidates what experience they have of the specific skill you are teaching and adapting your session accordingly. This means that on your instructor course you will not necessarily carry out a demonstration of the skill, but you must have checked the equipment beforehand so as not to inadvertently disadvantage the learners.

Explanation (Teach)

When teaching the skill, the instructor performs it, explaining what they are doing. During this phase it may be appropriate to engage candidates in helping with your explanation of the skill.

Practice (Facilitate)

This is where the majority of learning takes place. It should be by far the longest element of any skills session, as adults learn best when they are 'having a go' and are actively involved. Good support and encouragement during this stage is vital to facilitate independent practice of the skill. Where possible and appropriate, candidates should have more than one opportunity to practise.

Assessment (Assess)

If the skill is to be assessed fairly, candidates must perform it independently so that instructors can reach reliable decisions. Assessment might occur during facilitation or you may need a more formal approach to ensure that independent performance of the skill is assessed appropriately. To facilitate deep learning, the skills are then repeated and assessed to that same standard throughout the rest of the course.

Surface and deep learning

Simpson (1972) suggests skills development begins at a *surface* level, where the learner will require support, benefit from a focused environment and will learn by rote.

Deep learning can be seen in learners who explore and strive to interact with the content. They seek to relate, extend or transfer their knowledge of the topic and look to finding ways to contextualise it within their own work settings. Central to this approach is the need for instructors to provide feedback each time a candidate performs a skill. If we consider as an example suction skills, a 'deep' as opposed to 'surface' approach may be seen in the way in which we respond to a patient who has a complicated airway and is vomiting blood. Here the learner can modify what they are doing to create an improved outcome.

DeBourgh (2011) suggests that short skills practice, in a variety of situations and on multiple occasions, is the best way to create opportunities for deep learning. In practice, on life support courses, skills can be embedded *within* simulation sessions and instructors can ensure these continue to be practised to a high standard. Retention of skills is improved by their being used in different contexts and applied in different ways.

Interleaving, or mixing up the practice, whilst it may feel clumsy to the learner, has been shown by Brown et al. (2014) to increase learning. This is based on the notion of putting small barriers in the learner's way so that they have to work harder. This takes sensitivity to employ as an instructor as each student arrives at the session with a different history.

In a study using a spaced teaching approach, Patocka et al. (2015) taught bag and mask ventilation, intraosseous needle insertion and chest compressions. They concluded that learning skills over a longer period, with more opportunities for 'deliberate practice', increased the individual's ability to retain that knowledge.

> Deliberate practice *'is a highly structured activity, the explicit goal of which is to improve performance. Specific tasks are invented to overcome weaknesses, and performance is carefully monitored to provide cues for ways to improve it further.'*
>
> (Ericsson et al. 1993)

Caution is required on life support courses to avoid the risk that skills practice, for some, may never reach more than surface levels if candidates only learn by rote. We should therefore encourage them to continue to practise and use the skills as part of their continuing professional development.

Feedback can come from either the candidate themselves, other candidates or from instructors, providing opportunities for focused and specific practice. Digital feedback mechanisms continue to grow in popularity. Examples include chest compression feedback devices which provide data relating to depth, rate and recoil of chest compressions, providing immediate and objective feedback.

Rehearsal, repetition and feedback are critical elements of skills acquisition. Instructors need to correct errors and provide support to enable learners to carry out the skills correctly and enable them to develop appropriate muscle-memory.

Summary and learning

Good responsive skills teaching needs to be: hands-on, immersive and engaging.

Skills need to be taught in stages or steps - the number of steps will depend upon prior demonstration and explanation through online learning, practical experience, and the complexity of the skill.

Practice in a variety of contexts enhances learning.

Skills are most likely to be retained when deliberate practice, spaced practice and interleaving (mixing up the practice) is encouraged.

CHAPTER 6

Managing simulations

Introduction

Simulation has played an important role in clinical education for a number of years. Simulation teaching is based on the notion of a willing suspension of disbelief within which learners develop skills and behaviours, perhaps at the edge of their comfort zone. The benefits are felt not only by individuals, but by teams when training and working together. Through simulations, learners can build on their experiences in the work setting whether that be the ward, the Emergency Department or the out of hospital environment. Simulation is a widely used modality on life support courses and is particularly well placed for exploring non-technical skills (Chapter 12).

Pocket Guide to Teaching for Clinical Instructors, Fourth Edition.
Edited by Kate Denning, Kevin Mackie and Alan Charters, Andrew Lockey.
© 2025 John Wiley & Sons Ltd. Published 2025 by John Wiley & Sons Ltd.

> ## Learning outcomes
>
> This chapter will enable you to:
>
> - Assess the importance of simulated experiences within clinical education
> - Plan how to manage a simulation using a structured approach
> - Identify how simulation draws together learning from a number of contexts
> - Consider both physical and psychological safety in simulation

Simulation as a teaching modality

Eduardo Briceño (2016) describes how we can operate in the learning zone or the performance zone (Table 6.1). Both of these zones are essential, but our activities and intentions within them are different. At work, we are in the *performance zone* most of the time, with patients' lives at risk, making it unsafe to try out new approaches; therefore we use the *learning zone* to practise new skills and new approaches and to seek feedback in our lifelong goal of becoming better clinicians.

Table 6.1 Performance and learning zones

	Performance zone	Learning zone
Goal	Do the best we can	Improve
Activities for	Execution	Development
Concentrate on	Things I can already do	Things I haven't yet become skilled at
Mistakes	Minimised	Expected
Benefits	Immediate performance Getting things done	Growth and future performance

If we only ever 'perform', or get on with our jobs, we may work hard, but we will reach a plateau and will not improve as practitioners. It is important to move between the learning and performance zones so that we improve our performance and by doing so care for our patients more effectively. We achieve this by seeking feedback, by observing others, by reading around the subject and by implementing our new behaviours and skills during our next work shift.

The beauty of simulations is that they have the capacity to allow learners to operate within the learning zone and truly integrate both their experiences at work and their learning from other course elements. This capacity to bring together reading, pre-course e-learning, lectures, skills stations and workshops makes simulations central to most life support training. In something approaching real time, learners can interact with other health professionals and relevant equipment (e.g. monitors, tubes, fluids) and with manikins or actors. Simulation at its best has candidates engaging in a new/different experience in a safe and controlled setting where they are encouraged to explore, question, experiment, reflect and to compare their findings with their prior beliefs and experiences. They can then take what they have learned back to their work setting – their performance zone.

When we are learning with and from colleagues in a group setting, we are engaging in the social construction of learning, sometimes described as social constructivism. Simulation training epitomises this in a positive way and is often the part of the course that candidates enjoy the most, learning from others by observing their peers. There may be a focus on individual team members, though observers can also contribute to the debriefing process, to enhance reflection, to enable the development of strategies for improved performance and to build their own understanding of where the benchmarks of safe practice lie.

Simulation teaching differs from other teaching modalities in that, if successful, it relates directly to practice. It incorporates skills, knowledge and affect to enable learners to experiment within a safer version of their real world.

Realism

The impact of the intervention is enhanced if a high degree of realism can be maintained through accurate environmental and psychological simulation. An effective instructor can achieve high levels of realism through careful facilitation which can compensate for any lack of high-tech equipment. Environmental realism concerns *where* the simulation will be taking place and *what equipment* (or actors) will be used. Instructors will be required to adapt their facilitation and intervention depending on the degree of environmental realism that can be achieved.

The role of an embedded helper or participant instructor adds realism as information can be fed to the team/team leader from *within* the scenario. This contrasts with the slight contrivance of asking an instructor, who is operating outside the simulation, for clinical information.

Simple props such as having blankets available when exposing the patient or realistic patient notes can be affordable and effective ways of increasing the degree of realism. It can increase the candidates' cognitive load if we expect them to 'assume' that a piece of clinical equipment is in place. An example of this is having a simulated antibiotic infusion available if it is asked for.

Much of the psychological realism is premised on the fact that the clinical case being enacted is something that candidates might encounter in their working lives. As such, it has real significance for them and their practice.

A teaching structure: managing simulations

Prepare

Preparation includes checking the equipment, thinking about the layout and room temperature, an awareness of the need to avoid interruptions, and an in-depth knowledge of the scenario to be covered. Taking time to get these right is central to the success of the subsequent facilitation of the simulation.

Simulation can be delivered in quite diverse settings, including the classroom, a dedicated simulation suite or within the clinical environment. Careful consideration should be given to the most appropriate venue to ensure that proposed learning outcomes can be achieved.

Teaching rooms

Training centre: Life support courses often take place in training centres, using generic training facilities with lower fidelity manikins. If the simulation involves use of such a manikin, the responsibility for providing clinical information appropriately belongs to the instructor who is leading, or embedded within, the scenario. Instructors must prepare themselves so that they are familiar with the simulation and its likely progression.

Simulation suite: Many larger hospitals have a dedicated space for the delivery of simulation and debriefing, with suites supporting video recording or discrete observation facilities. The ability to simulate multiple clinical environments is also advantageous to heighten realism. Where a fully equipped simulation system is available, video-assisted debriefing can contribute a great deal. Using video-assistance takes training and experience but offers the potential for a powerful learning tool. Not least is the ability to supplement debriefing with playback of selected recordings. This can be particularly powerful when exploring situation awareness. Video playback can demonstrate how people react as information becomes available or may highlight moments of task fixation, possibly prompting a useful discussion on the role of communication in developing team awareness.

The impact of leadership and communication style can also be demonstrated with video. It is common for people to feel anxious during simulated practice, and video can be used to show how they remained outwardly controlled. Similarly, if a team leader issues instructions that are untargeted or vague, then the team's response might be highlighted and reflected upon. However, video is rarely used in life support courses because of time constraints and availability of suitable equipment.

Clinical area: More portable medium/high fidelity manikins can be used to support simulation within a clinical environment, in what is sometimes described as in situ simulation training. Clearly the most significant barrier to this form of learning is the lack of appropriate time and space within a setting, where real patients may inadvertently observe and be confused by some part of the simulation.

In situ training has the added benefit of developing increased fidelity by using existing personnel, equipment and other resources directly from clinical areas. In some cases, learning alongside colleagues provides reassurance, though it may also result in increased anxiety; this can be alleviated by careful pre-briefing, in order to create an accessible learning environment. Such in situ simulations fit into the category that Briceño (2016) describes as 'low stakes islands' within the high stakes setting of the performance zone, places where learning can be unexpected and/or significant and where changes can be made relatively swiftly.

Equipment

Whether the simulation is low or high fidelity it is the instructors' duty to check that the equipment is working as required. This means arriving well before the learners, checking the equipment, and then agreeing with colleagues which roles each of you will take and how much time you have for each section of the session (briefing, running the simulation, debriefing). Instructors are expected to be knowledgeable about the simulation narrative and to have a good idea of how to respond if a candidate behaves unexpectedly. Although paperwork is provided and is helpful, it cannot answer all of a candidate's questions.

Actors or patients can be used to enhance a simulation where invasive emergency treatments are not required. Among the difficulties presented by real patients or actors is the need to behave realistically; they will need to be carefully briefed and must rehearse the simulation so that difficulties can be resolved.

Simulation does not always require highly realistic manikins, tabletop exercises can still encourage sufficient interaction between people to draw out useful learning.

Technology-enhanced simulation

Within this simulation modality the instructor can control the pre-recorded responses of an on-screen patient (avatar) guiding the simulation based on the candidate's interactions and responses. The instructor can respond to the degree of anxiety demonstrated by the candidate to ensure safety is maintained. Technology-enhanced simulation for mass training might pose logistical problems for life support courses. Future advances in augmented and virtual reality may mean that there is potential for their use in our courses, but this would need careful management to ensure that the operation of technology does not detract from learning.

Open

When opening a simulation session, the instructor should make clear the purpose of the simulation, including learning outcomes. At the heart of simulation teaching is role play, in which learners act out how to behave in a clinical case. In the case of learners on life support courses, the expectation is that the role they play is that of themselves. In other words, they improvise actions based on their usual behaviour but in a novel context. As an instructor, you should aspire to make the simulations as real as possible to maximise the learning experience for everyone.

Careful pre-briefing of the candidates is essential to ensure that all participants are clear on their roles, learning outcomes and on the expectations of the faculty. This may be an opportunity to advise candidates of any defective equipment or problems with the manikin. Rudolph et al. (2014) suggest that an effective briefing prior to a simulation can create a space for learners to be more open to taking risks, operating outside of their comfort zone and receiving and acting on feedback.

Simulations may provoke anxiety for both learners and instructors. Candidates may fear performing in front of colleagues, with the additional pressure of continuous assessment. Stressing that the scenario is taking place in the learning zone, *not* the performance zone, can be helpful. For faculty there is the anxiety of managing multiple factors to enable the simulation to run smoothly. Candidates may arrive with limited or negative experiences of simulation, which can impact on how they experience the current episode. It is important to recognise any physical and psychological responses resulting from increased anxiety or confusion, and the impact this may have on learning. The instructor plays a critical role in managing anxiety and maintaining safety, to ensure the candidates achieve their potential. This is discussed in more detail in Chapter 7.

Candidates who have a lot of experience of simulation and have accustomed themselves to the approach are able to buy-in to the notion of 'pretending' that the manikin is a child or adult in need of their care. For others the notion of role play is enough to put them off the learning event altogether. Facilitators must empathise with this problem and treat it as normal. Strategies to help these candidates include:

- Avoiding use of the phrase role play
- Locating the scenario within a familiar setting for the candidate
- Suggesting a name for the patient to enhance the bond
- Encouraging them to say out loud what they are thinking

Practicalities of positioning the group of candidates, expectations of individuals and their level of involvement should all be clearly explained in the briefing. You should also be clear about timings of the session and explain that when you stop in order to debrief, this need not be a reflection on how well the candidate has managed the event.

Facilitate

During the facilitation phase, candidates should be presented with the specific clinical scenario they will be managing. This briefing should accurately replicate a request for assistance and could use an SBAR/ISBARD format or other communication method used locally.

Example briefing

Identification	I am X, the patient is X and I am talking with X
Situation	55-year-old male, 2-hour history of chest pain
Background	Known ischaemic heart disease, takes nitrate and beta-blockers
Assessment	RR 24, HR 110 irregular, BP 180/100
Recommendation	Immediately request full assessment and further investigations
Decision	Agree to attend. Please take 12-lead ECG, establish cardiac monitoring and arrange chest x-ray

The instructor must allow an opportunity for candidates to ask questions in order to clarify key points before they commence the simulation. It is also useful to get them to repeat the outline of the case, to reassure both them and you that they have understood. Encouraging teams to find a moment to plan and prepare for activities can be very helpful and aligns with the preparations made in clinical practice.

As the simulation progresses there are times when the instructor needs to clarify points and ask questions. This should be limited as it will impact on realism and may turn the simulation into a discussion between the instructor and candidate.

Some life support courses advocate 'time outs' to encourage team leaders to discuss their approach or their uncertainties with their team. These can be extremely valuable as a way of involving the rest of the group, but should be used judiciously.

Whilst treating a patient in a simulation the team leader may do something unexpected. Your response to this will be guided by multiple factors such as the anxiety levels of the candidate and the impact of the intervention or omission on patient safety. Consider the range of possible responses below:

> **Example responses**
>
> Candidate fails to apply high flow oxygen to a septic patient with saturations of 88%
>
> **Possible response:** Drop the saturations further, add an audible low saturations alarm. Remind the candidate that the monitor will give an alarm
>
> **Possible response from embedded faculty helper:** *'It looks as if the patient is becoming paler, is there anything you'd like me to do?'*
>
> **Possible response:** Bring in other team members to make suggestions relating to the required actions
>
> **Possible response:** *'Can you tell me what you are thinking at the moment? Your team may be able to help you'*

If a candidate is becoming too anxious the instructor must take actions to alleviate this. Buchanan and Huczynski (2013) describe 'arousal states' in learners. Too much or too little intervention can raise anxiety levels to a point where performance is severely affected. A degree of emotional intelligence is essential to gauge what impact your interventions are having on your learner/s.

Where the simulation is taking place in a dedicated simulation facility, the faculty may be present in a separate room. Additional support can be 'parachuted' into the simulation to provide subtle guidance to a struggling team.

During simulations there may be opportunities to enhance realism and thereby increase understanding. Consider this example:

Example conversation

Candidate to instructor: *'What's the blood pressure?'*

Instructor: *'You have a helper, and there's equipment on the resuscitation trolley'*

Candidate: *'Oh yes, could you check the blood pressure please?'*

Instructor: *'The blood pressure is 90/35'*

It may also be possible to show the blood pressure on a monitor along with other vital signs, or an embedded faculty member could 'whisper' the information to another team member so that they can give the information to assist the team leader's decision making. The Advanced Paediatric Life Support (APLS) and European Trauma Course (ETC) make use of 'whispering' and cue cards to provide relevant clinical information from within the simulation.

When something unexpected happens, your first priority is to maintain the safety (physical and psychological) of those present so occasionally this may require you to terminate the simulation. Where safety has *not* been impacted, efforts should be made to maintain the simulation's fidelity: the learning outcomes can often still be achieved by altering the course of the simulation slightly.

Another responsibility for instructors is to manage the flow of time. Some learners may need to be prompted by adding in new, and possibly urgent, clinical signs (e.g. *'The patient is losing consciousness'*). Other team members can be brought in to offer support and suggestions. Others may move rapidly, often by telling the instructor a list of what needs to be done, rather than actually doing it. The latter can be controlled by simple requests, for example:

Example conversation

Learner: *'I would insert two IV lines, measure capillary refill and take the blood pressure'*

Instructor: *'Show me how you would make sure those tasks are completed'*

Remember, the simulation is intended to integrate skills and knowledge acquired elsewhere; learners may need to be encouraged to demonstrate their psychomotor ability as well as their knowledge.

During the simulation itself, the instructor is there to provide clinical signs or triggers (where necessary), prompt (if required), listen and manage time boundaries. How this is achieved will depend on the equipment used (verbally in a low fidelity setting or through the manikin during higher fidelity simulations) and whether or not the instructor is embedded or operating outside the simulation.

The simulation can be finished by:

- Bringing in an appropriate expert and asking the team leader to handover
- Asking the team leader what they felt was happening or what they would like to do next
- Simply saying, '*Thank you, we'll end it there*'

The next phase of the learning, in the form of the debrief, can then begin. In this stage candidates will be encouraged to 'return to normal' after the simulation, which allows them to step back from the experience and begin to analyse it from 'outside'. It is really helpful to move away from the simulation to emphasise this shift.

An effective, learner-centred debrief will support the whole group's learning by encouraging reflection and identifying strategies for improvement. National and international resuscitation courses use the learning conversation to explore key issues, as discussed in Chapter 8. However, as courses move towards a model of continuous assessment, the debrief should also ensure that candidates know whether they have performed to the required standard. Skills are often assessed throughout the course, so if a candidate within the team does not perform to the required standard this should be addressed during the debrief. Examples might include unsafe defibrillation or poor quality chest compressions that need to be identified and remedied as necessary.

Close

As we have seen in this chapter, simulation will have a strong emotional component that will resonate with candidates' own clinical practice. For example, conducting a simulation involving challenging conversations related to suicide may be triggering for those who have experienced this trauma either personally or from clinical practice. This may mean the mentor offering support, or helping individuals to find additional support elsewhere.

The session may have included more than one simulation; therefore it is important to invite questions or comments to resolve issues that have emerged during the entire session. Note that 'any questions' is not an extension of the debrief.

A brief summary of *key* learning points which have been identified during the session will be useful. It may be as simple as:

Example summary

'*This morning you have seen how sepsis can be managed effectively, with particular emphasis on identifying relevant reversible causes. We also discussed the importance of closing the communication loop when requesting interventions, especially when you are the team leader.*'

Simulations form the heart of most life support courses and often pose the most challenges to us as instructors. However, when they are facilitated with sensitivity and good structure they can be rewarding, immersive and enjoyable for instructors and learners alike.

Summary and learning

Simulation is a highly effective tool in clinical education.

It allows candidates to apply theory, skills, and behaviours in a realistic scenario firmly located in the learning zone, enabling them to act more effectively in the performance zone when they return to work.

To enhance learning, candidates should be able to relate the simulation to their own clinical area through the maintenance of realism and fidelity.

The use of effective debriefing is an important part of the experiential learning cycle, enabling reflection and the development of strategies for improved performance.

Since simulation can evoke a strong emotional response, the instructor must understand and acknowledge such reactions with empathy.

CHAPTER 7

Psychological safety

Introduction

As instructors, we should be aware that factors such as learning from errors, patient safety and concerns about career progression may increase stress for candidates. Add to these the pressure of performing in front of colleagues, being continuously assessed and personal difficulties and we can easily understand why some candidates may feel uneasy, thus limiting their ability to learn. In this chapter we consider what may drive such responses and see how the instructor can develop a safer learning space.

Learning outcomes

This chapter will enable you to:

- Explain the sympathetic and parasympathetic systems
- Identify how to support candidates' wellbeing
- Create a psychologically safe learning environment
- Recognise the impact of mindset and imposter syndrome, and review methods of mitigating these problems

Pocket Guide to Teaching for Clinical Instructors, Fourth Edition.
Edited by Kate Denning, Kevin Mackie and Alan Charters, Andrew Lockey.
© 2025 John Wiley & Sons Ltd. Published 2025 by John Wiley & Sons Ltd.

Threat, drive and soothe

One way of conceptualising how we regulate our emotions is to think in terms of three states, described by Gilbert (2009) as 'threat', 'drive' and 'soothe'. Figure 7.1 illustrates these three systems, how they interact with each other and the emotions contained within each of them.

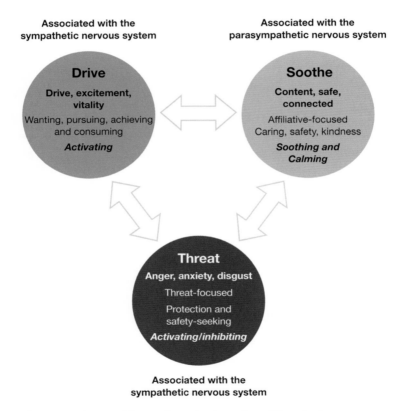

Figure 7.1 Threat, drive and soothe based on Gilbert's three system model

The three system model illustrates how our evolutionary journey has shaped our emotional responses, because our predominant need has historically been to keep ourselves physically safe (Irons and Beaumont, 2017). It is helpful to bear this in mind when making sense of how our emotional, physical and behavioural responses are linked. It can also give us a greater understanding of why we, and those around us, are sometimes triggered to have seemingly disproportionate responses.

Emotional responses are driven by the autonomic nervous system, which comprises two antagonistic parts: the sympathetic (fight or flight) and the parasympathetic (rest and digest) nervous systems (Figure 7.2). A sympathetic response is activated when we are under threat and our body prepares for action; a parasympathetic response uses less energy and signals that the body is entering a calm state.

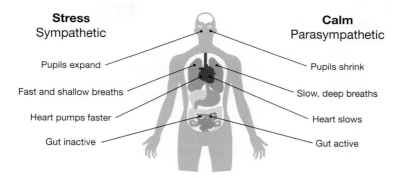

Figure 7.2 Sympathetic and parasympathetic nervous system

The sympathetic nervous system: threat and drive

A 'threat' response is a call to action, activated by potential or actual danger (fight, flight or freeze), and causing physical reactions such as increased heart rate, dilated pupils, perspiration and muscle tension.

It can also be activated by memories of previous experiences. Irons and Beaumont (2017) explain that stressful, painful or frightening situations can make us wary and anxious, determined to 'keep our head down' in the future. This response can manifest itself as a general lack of engagement, which to the observer may appear to be antipathy towards the learning process (see following box).

Example responses

A candidate becomes extremely concerned when asked to take part in a simulation. They recall feeling ridiculed during a debrief following an error and are apprehensive that this will happen again.

Possible response: A clear pre-briefing before the simulation will help. It should emphasise how the team is likely to make mistakes, an important element of working within the learning zone. Candidate roles and responsibilities should be clarified.

Possible response: Be alert to candidates' demeanour so that you can pick up this type of hesitancy. Then proceed with empathy and ensure that you listen to their perspective, encourage any tentative steps at learning, and avoid giving your own examples/stories which will only be a distraction.

The 'drive' system, the sympathetic response, motivates us to get things done, makes social connections and creates a sense of achievement. Dopamine, a reward chemical, is released from the brain, encouraging the person to continue seeking further reward. The drive system can be a positive influence, but if it continues for prolonged periods, giving the person no opportunity to restore and recharge, it can cause problems (see following box). Counter-intuitively, remaining in this state can also lead to procrastination and depleted motivation.

Remaining in a threat or drive state, with the sympathetic nervous system on high alert for long periods of time, can significantly affect mental and physical health. For instance, healthcare professionals, working long hours under stress, may feel that they have no choice but to carry on despite difficulties, and always be there for patients and colleagues. This traditional attitude, however, implies that a professional's wellbeing is of secondary importance to the demands of the service. Instructors can help learners

Example responses

A highly motivated candidate arrives after completing several long days in a busy Emergency Department.

Possible response: Mentors should check in with all their mentees to ensure they are OK. In this particular instance you are looking to see that the candidate has the physical and emotional reserves to be able to benefit from attendance on the course.

Possible response: Give the candidate the opportunity to restore and recharge as far as you are able by encouraging them either to talk or to have quiet time during refreshment breaks.

Possible response: Make sure that other members of the faculty are aware of the potential difficulties this may create for the candidate. Remaining vigilant to their mental state can be extremely helpful, but is also a courtesy which we can extend to all of our colleagues.

to find more effective behaviours by making sensible choices for their own wellbeing and by discouraging the sort of stoicism that leads to burn out.

The parasympathetic nervous system

The 'soothe' system creates a parasympathetic response, restoring emotional equilibrium so that we are able to calm down and think more clearly. The soothe system releases chemicals such as endorphins and oxytocin. Welford (2016) explains that when we find ourselves in this state, or consciously choose to switch it on, the threat and drive states are switched off. The soothe system can be initiated by an individual but, more importantly to us here, the instructor may also enable its initiation, or at least provide suitable opportunities and space for it to happen (see following box).

Example responses

A candidate appears increasingly anxious about being the team leader in a simulation.

Possible response: Find ways to activate the candidate's soothe system by, for example, talking the group through a simple box-breathing exercise (Figure 7.3).

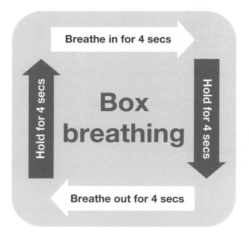

Figure 7.3 Box breathing exercise

Van der Kolk (2014) suggests that despite the well-documented effects of anger, fear and anxiety on the ability to reason, many continue to ignore the need to engage the safety system of the brain before trying to promote new ways of thinking. In a heightened emotional state, capacity to focus is diminished. The threat system response is powerful, designed to keep us safe; thus, even when we know what might be helpful to mediate this response, it can be very difficult to put it into action because the brain's response is 'better safe than sorry'.

Instructors have a number of ways to improve psychological safety (Figure 7.4) and ensure that risks are taken without fear of significant personal consequence.

Actions	How this might look
Ensure a friendly and warm welcome	Candidates must feel valued and respected. Demonstrate that you are interested in every person in the group
Create a safe environment	Instructors should make sure not only that the course is a safe place in which to learn but that the candidates are all assured that it is so
Build rapport at an early stage	How you do this will be unique to you. Some people do it with humour; others are exceptionally good at listening and drawing people out. If you can find something in each candidate to respond to on a personal level they will appreciate it
Respond positively to mistakes	Candidates need to **know** that they are free to take risks and make mistakes; they provide opportunities for the group to learn, and prove that they are stretching themselves
Identify the signs of anxiety and threat early	Be alert to signs that candidates are shutting down. Modify your approach, give candidates space and time if needed. In extreme situations stop the interaction and provide appropriate emotional support
Demonstrate your own vulnerability	This can help to develop connections between instructors and candidates
Ensure support is available	Ensure that time for discussion of concerns is available away from the learning environment. Valuable support for instructors and learners can be provided by course and medical directors
Be explicit and clear	Ensure all candidates are aware of the mechanisms in place to support their safety. Know what external support candidates can access for more profound issues
Treat all colleagues with respect	Instructors do not set out to humiliate learners, but being on the receiving end of feedback is very different from giving it. Also, consider your role in respecting co-instructors, administrative support staff and course directors

Figure 7.4 Enhancing psychological safety

Imposter syndrome

'Imposter syndrome' is a psychological term for feelings of doubt in one's own abilities and anxiety about being exposed as a fraud, even in those who are outwardly successful. It is a chronic sense of inadequacy, not meeting others' expectations and/or not being at the same standard as one's peers.

Those who suffer badly from imposter syndrome are more likely to be women, people of colour and those from ethnic minorities. Despite reports suggesting that the syndrome decreases with age, it actually occurs in men and women of all ages. Those who self-report difficulties in managing their work–life balance are also much more likely to report symptoms of imposter syndrome, which may be exacerbated by caring responsibilities, financial stressors and other factors such as anxiety and depression.

Recently, opinions on imposter syndrome have shifted, with writers questioning whether the label is overused and whether it masks systemic issues of racial and gender bias. As Mullangi and Jagsi (2019) say, is it surprising that someone feels like an imposter when they do not fit a specific workplace demographic.

The problem with imposter syndrome as a concept is that it puts the blame, and the locus of control, on individuals, without accounting for the historical and cultural contexts from which it springs. It *pathologises* a feeling of discomfort, inadequacy and, possibly, second-guessing the cultural norms, which are all very common feelings (Tulshyan and Burey, 2021).

That being said, in your teaching careers you will still come across a number of people who will display or talk about these feelings, or who will freely use the label 'impostor syndrome'.

Many strategies are suggested to help, though few of these are evidence-based. One such suggestion is to acknowledge the person's feelings and ensure that they feel safe enough to discuss them. By letting them know that these feelings of inadequacy are real, and very common, you can help them feel less alone. Talking openly about this in a group setting can encourage others to share their coping strategies and empower someone to view things in a different and more rewarding way.

Challenging self-criticism with empirical evidence can be of more help than platitudes or vague niceties. For example, if the learner is concerned that they have 'no right' to be on a Generic Instructor Course (GIC), remind them of the selection process and statistics, and encourage them to 'let go of perfectionism'. However, perfectionism is closely linked to patient safety and letting go of it must be considered with caution *in the clinical setting*.

Feelings of inadequacy can be crippling to both learners and mentors, but acknowledging these feelings in a sensitive way can help reassure candidates. Instructors should try to create an atmosphere that addresses and acknowledges systemic bias and racism.

Mindset: growth and fixed

As a mentor, you will find it helpful to have an awareness of the candidates' (**and your own**) mindset, aspects of which are characterised as 'growth' or 'fixed' (Figure 7.5). Those who believe they will progress through hard work, feedback and discovery of new strategies are said to have a growth mindset. Those who believe their talents to be innate and immutable are said to possess a fixed mindset (Dweck, 2006).

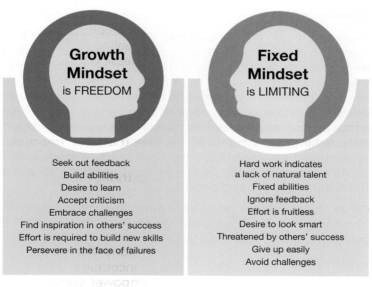

Figure 7.5 Growth or fixed mindset

This deceptively simple explanation masks some complexities because our mindset is affected by different contexts. Learners who feel scared, unsafe, disinterested, attacked or overwhelmed may veer towards the 'fixed' end of the continuum. In another time and place, these same people will display characteristics of a 'growth' mindset.

Growth mindset

When operating with a growth mindset we tend to value learning and embrace mistakes as part of the process, since making mistakes and learning from others helps us develop new strategies for improvement. It is particularly evident after a clinical simulation, where during the debrief individuals engage fully with the process, and mistakes are considered as opportunities for development.

To encourage a growth mindset you might ask learners to come up with multiple different approaches to a problem, to turn to their team for ideas and support, to tell themselves they will soon be able to achieve what at present seems impossible, and to remember that expert advice is available and it is good to seek it out.

Fixed mindset

The person who has slipped into a fixed mindset will fear making mistakes, do anything to avoid them and respond negatively to feedback, which is seen as a criticism of them as a person rather than their actions. This can be seen in high-risk industries, such as healthcare, where mistakes can have disastrous consequences. It may also occur on our courses, where personal career progression is at stake. During a debrief, if a candidate demonstrates reluctance to accept that they have made mistakes and offers excuses for poor performance, this *may* indicate a fixed mindset in that moment.

Other clues to this mindset lie in remarks such as 'I can't do technology', 'I've never been good at maths' or 'I'm a paediatric nurse, I don't do trauma'.

We can all succumb to a fixed mindset when things do not go to plan, when someone criticises our efforts, when we feel unsafe and when we begin to compare ourselves unfavourably with others.

What can instructors do to help mindset issues?

- Ensure a psychologically safe space for learning (Figure 7.4)
- Encourage candidates to 'have a go'
- Acknowledge the difficulties and the discomfort
- Focus on the process
- Be aware that ongoing assessment can be stressful for candidates
- Listen and acknowledge candidates' concerns
- Avoid making assumptions
- Focus on whatever progress is being made
- Explain how and why you are using particular manikins or equipment
- Encourage the group to seek alternative approaches
- Provide opportunities away from the group to reflect on feelings and experience

As instructors, it is important that we have an awareness of how mindset can influence learning (and the experience of learning) for us and our candidates. Avoid 'labelling' candidates as this pushes them towards a fixed mindset. For example, suppose you were told as a child that you were the sporty one and your sister was the clever one, this would affect your self-image for a long time. Thus, in the context of a life support course, rather than telling a candidate that they need to be more confident (an almost impossible task) it is more helpful to give them concrete, useful behaviours to practise (growth mindset).

Compare:

'*You need to be more confident*'

with:

'*Consider the tone and pace of your delivery*'

or

'*Next time have a go at speaking a bit slower/ louder and see what effect that has*'

Summary and learning

A psychologically safe space for learning is essential.

Understanding the threat, drive, soothe response allows instructors to maintain safety and enable candidates to operate effectively.

Recognition of feelings of inadequacy, and the effects of mindset can make us more supportive of our candidates.

CHAPTER 8

Debriefing as a learning conversation

Introduction

In the world of clinical education, debriefing is considered the most important feature of simulation. It allows learners to reflect on the simulated teaching event and to use what they have learned to improve their practice, as per Kolb's experiential learning cycle (Chapter 1). In order to be effective, the process of debrief needs to be sensitive, relevant and useful: the challenge is to find the appropriate language.

Feedback for learners occurs in different ways during life support courses; in pre-course learning, skills teaching, assessment and simulations. It is a *component* of any debrief but should not be its entirety.

> ## Learning outcomes
>
> This chapter will enable you to:
> - Define debrief and its contribution to learning
> - Formulate responsive feedback
> - Consider the components of a useful learning conversation

Pocket Guide to Teaching for Clinical Instructors, Fourth Edition.
Edited by Kate Denning, Kevin Mackie and Alan Charters, Andrew Lockey.
© 2025 John Wiley & Sons Ltd. Published 2025 by John Wiley & Sons Ltd.

Debriefing

Debrief has gone through several discrete phases in recent years, emphasising first results, then raising self-esteem and more recently focusing on collaborative dialogue. Debriefing in life support courses has, for a number of years, concentrated on the latter, using an approach that is conversational in nature, with input from both instructors and learners. This chapter will explore how to get the best out of this collaborative, dialogic approach.

An approach based on conversation, or discussion, has significant advantages. Saunders and Gowing (1999) found that learners favoured '*a mutual discussion of the work rather than [being] exposed to one-sided evaluation and criticism*', while Juwah et al. (2004) wrote '*External feedback as a transmission process involving "telling" ignores the active role the learner must play in constructing meaning from feedback messages*'. In other words, students need to play a central role in identifying their own learning.

Debriefing as a learning conversation

A learning conversation has two broad strands (Figure 8.1): first you need to elicit and explore issues that the learner identifies; after this you can raise an issue that you have noticed, but the learner did not mention, and explore this.

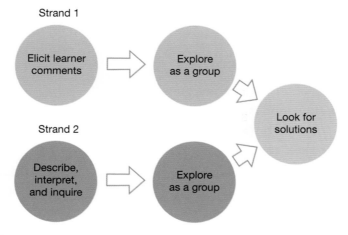

Figure 8.1 Overview of the learning conversation (Davis and Denning, 2018)

With both strands it is crucial to include the perceptions and perspectives of the rest of the group, and to allow them to reach solutions to any questions or problems that arise.

> Consider this as a loose structure, for, as Carr (2006), writes: '*It is important that a variety of different techniques are used and that the approach be varied each time so the experience does not become predictable.*'

The issue of predictability has been raised by learners commenting on highly structured debriefs that they have experienced. In contrast, a well-managed and authentic learning conversation leaves candidates feeling valued and clear about their next steps. A genuine conversation is not at risk of becoming predictable because it responds to the learner's agenda.

The learning conversation has been designed with tight time constraints in mind. When used effectively, it is focused, economical and supportive because of the lack of redundancy and a direct focus on thoughts voiced by learners. The elements are shown in Figure 8.2 and described in detail below.

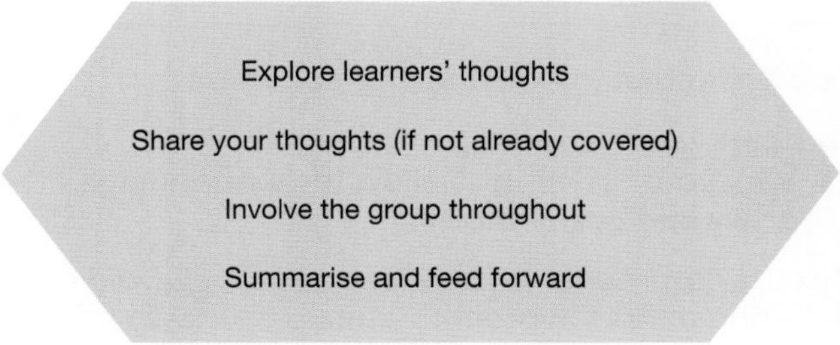

Explore learners' thoughts

Share your thoughts (if not already covered)

Involve the group throughout

Summarise and feed forward

Figure 8.2 Learning conversation

Starting the conversation

In starting the conversation, the facilitator is looking to find out what the learner wants to discuss. Sometimes this happens spontaneously. On other occasions learners wait for the facilitator to initiate the conversation. In this case, it is important that the facilitator uses a phrase that is authentic to their conversational style and allows for the learner to also respond authentically.

Start the learning conversation

- *'What did that simulation feel like?'*
- *'Is there anything you would like to explore from that simulation?'*
- *'How was that?'*
- Silence or non-verbal cue

The learner's initial reaction to the conversation opener is usually the thought that is uppermost in their minds. Often this is the one small error that they made in an otherwise good practice. However positive the instructor feels about the overall performance, it is important to listen and acknowledge these tensions as being key to the candidate's own experience. They may not be receptive to further conversation without having first shared their own thoughts and feelings. On occasions they may need to talk through the whole experience to make sense of it. Time constraints, however, mean that you can usually only concentrate on the key aspects of the simulation.

Good practice in starting the conversation

- Start with a short, open question
- Vary your opening to allow for authenticity and avoid predictability

Discuss comments as they are made and avoid deferring a topic in order to pursue your own agenda

Exploring the learner's thoughts

An exploration of the learner's thoughts should follow seamlessly on from the start of the conversation. This phase should feature two essential elements: open-ended questions and the use of silence. Learners have many ideas and profound insight if we give them time to formulate and express their thoughts. If instructors verbalise *for* learners we deprive them of the possibility of being exploratory and reflective, hence the need to stop talking and let silence work. For the learning conversation to be effective, it needs to be reactive, not pre-prepared, which means listening in a way that notes all potential signals, including non-verbal communication.

You may have heard facilitators make frequent use of examples from their own experience: comments such as *'When I get into that situation I find it useful to. . .'*. This may be helpful to the learner but it is crucial not to overwhelm them with your own personal experience when they are still deeply involved with their own recent learning event. As a facilitator, you should spend more time listening than talking – often much more of a challenge than it sounds.

Effective listening occurs when the facilitator focuses on the learner with genuine interest, not being distracted by working out what they themselves are going to say next. It will also help if you are comfortable with silence and possess a non-hierarchical model of learning, a belief that others may have a perspective that will enlighten the situation. Throughout the learning conversation, maintaining a global vigilance and processing non-verbal as well as verbal communication will create a wider channel of understanding.

Good practice in exploring ideas

- Listen intently and deal with any thoughts as they arise through including the group
- Clarify any discussion points that may be misinterpreted, drawing on the group's knowledge and experiences
- Allow the discussion to flow naturally
- Keep focused on the candidate or team's performance, avoiding anecdotes or 'handy hints'
- Listen to understand, not to respond
- Avoid the temptation to rush the discussion of learner's thoughts if they do not synchronise with what you want to talk about

Including the group

Low fidelity simulation is increasingly viewed as a group event with members either being part of the team assisting during the simulation, or observing. The conversation can, and should, involve the group in sharing their perspective of anything they thought particularly pertinent. Consider Figure 8.3 in which the facilitator is marked in red, the team leader in blue and other group members in green.

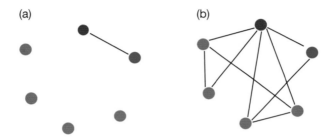

Figure 8.3 (a, b) Facilitation styles during debrief

Figure 8.3a shows what has been described as 'verbal ping pong' (Askew and Lodge, 2000) between the facilitator and the learner which excludes other members of the group: this practice should be avoided in most situations. Figure 8.3b shows the conversation as a web where the conversation sometimes goes through the facilitator but not always; the facilitator is vigilant but not dominant, has control but is not controlling. This is what we are aiming for with the learning conversation.

Perhaps the best way to ensure group involvement is to resist responding to the learner yourself. You do not need to look disinterested, merely to leave spaces, to use non-verbal cues or to offer the learner's question back for the group to respond. You can also include the group by asking questions of individuals or of everyone.

Examples of questions to involve the group

- 'What was the main clinical issue here?'
- [to the team] 'How did you see your role in the simulation?'
- 'How do you make sure you remember the drug doses when at work?'
- 'What alternatives can anyone suggest for that difficult situation?'

Debrief should involve discussion amongst a group of peers to enhance everyone's understanding of the technical and clinical issues that emerged in the content of the simulation. It should also provide space to explore non-technical issues and consider alternative behaviours to practise in future simulations.

What we should avoid is asking the group to give the learner difficult feedback that we ourselves do not want to give. Significant problems should be pointed out by the instructor, as discussed in the next section.

Sharing your thoughts

In some settings, only a few minutes are allocated to the debrief, in which case it is important not to waste time by reiterating comments already made. Not only is this unnecessary, but it also undermines the recent discussion. Equally you do not have time, or indeed need, to list the learner's achievements, even though you may wish to raise their esteem. It is more effective to highlight one or two key points, either as strengths or as areas for improvement. Candidates will probably be unable to absorb a long list of achievements, anyway.

Making a few notes during a simulation will help remind yourself of any specific feedback you would like to give. If appropriate, write down a person's actual words to avoid paraphrasing, or 'interpreting', which may be misleading.

When raising something that has not yet been discussed, we need to consider how to do so in a way that encourages learning rather than raising defensiveness. The approach used increasingly, but not exclusively, in simulation centres is 'advocacy with inquiry' which has its origins in action science (Argyris et al., 1985). This method has come to the attention of practitioners of low and high fidelity simulation through the process described as 'debriefing with good judgement' (see, for example, Rudolph et al., 2007). Broadly speaking, when you want to raise a point for discussion you should do so with genuine inquiry. Start by providing the facts (i.e. describe what you have noticed, being as specific as your recall allows). You may also add your own *interpretation* of what happened, acknowledging that you have a perspective (we all have our own biases and tend to favour our own interpretation); then seek clarification from the learner about their perspective, or give them the opportunity to explain their rationale for acting as they did.

Your comments should be *descriptive*, focused on the behaviours you have witnessed. If you say '*You started resuscitating the patient too late*', you may get more of a defensive response than '*It felt to me that there were a few seconds lag between handover and you starting resuscitation, can you tell me more about that?*' Presenting your observations as judgement or assumption may encourage the learner to shut down, feel embarrassed and not engage further with the process of learning. Obviously, this is best avoided. Equally it is unhelpful to be truly non-judgemental in your learning conversation, as this denies the fact that you have a perspective. Instead, debriefing with *good* judgement (Rudolph et al., 2007) allows us to focus on the learning whilst also allowing candidates to feel safe and able to learn and make changes.

The key here is to describe the candidate's behaviour: for example '*When you were checking the circulation you asked for a blood pressure reading and for the monitors to be put on*'. It can then be helpful, as indicated above, to acknowledge that you (the observer) have a perspective on this. For example, '*I wasn't sure who this was directed at*'. Having clarified your own thought process, the next step is to ask the learner to respond in kind. For example, the question '*Can you recall what was going on from your perspective at that moment?*' Advocacy with inquiry is a useful technique to avoid 'guess what teacher's thinking' questions which often mask a hidden agenda.

In summary, it is particularly effective to describe what we have seen and to encourage learners to explore their actions and, if appropriate, identify alternative behaviours. They are then more likely to retain the knowledge, having played a full part in the discussion and in finding the solution.

Advocacy with inquiry is sometimes described in rather rigid terms but in reality, and in order to sound natural, it takes many forms. Some examples showing different approaches to raising difficult issues are:

- At that point I thought X was going on, *what did you think was happening?*
- When the patient collapsed it took you 2 minutes to initiate CPR and I was starting to get worried. *What was going through your mind at the time?*
- I am wondering if ... *does this sound like a possibility?*
- I noticed that you put the oxygen on during your assessment of circulation; *can you tell me what prompted you to do that?*
- During the simulation I gave you a bit of a hint about glucose and you looked frustrated with yourself that you'd forgotten it. *What are your thoughts on strategies for remembering it in future?*

When discussing specific incidents or occurrences it may be helpful to think in the following terms

- What did I see? (and give a description of this, being as accurate as possible)
- How did I interpret this? (acknowledge that I have a perspective)
- Am I missing something? (be open to a range of responses rather than anticipating just one)

Remaining learner-centred

The moment the facilitator stops trying to force the learner into their frame and shows interest in the learner's frame, acknowledging their constraints as real, it becomes possible for learning and change to occur. Everyone in the room can learn when the conversation is approached with genuine interest. An awareness of your own frame and how that might affect your approach will help you better understand what influence you may inadvertently be applying.

Learners are vulnerable during debrief and sometimes feel unwilling to enter into a prolonged conversation. It is easy, from the outside, to see a host of errors, and to give a lot of negative information, which is not helpful. Facilitators should be aware of this and use empathy to acknowledge that from the learner's perspective the situation might be difficult, stressful or embarrassing. Some level of emotional understanding will enhance the learning process. Empathy may also mean deciding to withhold or defer some of your observations.

When a candidate has really struggled, you may find the debrief challenging because of an innate desire to be positive. There are two issues here. The first is about maintaining our integrity, since learners may find it hard to trust an instructor who, trying to remain positive, has been less than truthful. And the second is that we must ensure that learning occurs, that errors are corrected and that the learner is in a frame of mind to be able to listen, evaluate, interact and suggest alternative strategies.

Ways to ensure learning during a challenging debrief

- Appreciate the learner's feelings and desire to improve
- Acknowledge the learner's own perception of errors and any helpful suggestions they may have for improvement
- Listen attentively to the learners, support them and show that you value their personal reflections
- See issues as learning opportunities, rather than negatives
- Be alert to the negative impact of unnecessarily repeating challenging feedback

Checking for unresolved issues and summarising

As you move towards the end of the learning conversation, check whether anyone else has ideas that could help the group increase their understanding and progress. This is not asking for questions (as in the teaching session), it is merely making sure that all relevant and pertinent points have been covered. Include the team leader, the rest of the group and the other instructor in the room; however, the other instructor should not routinely contribute here. The intention at this stage is simply to deal with anything that has not already been covered. Candidates are often positive in their support of the team leader who tends to be at the centre of the debrief. We should not underestimate the importance of this: it has value in terms of building confidence, group cohesion and self-esteem.

Keep the summary brief to avoid repeating points that were made only a short time ago. It can be very useful to ask the candidate to summarise the discussion by asking them how they are going to rectify any performance deficits. If time allows, the group can also be asked to think about how their own practice may be improved.

Once the debrief has finished, avoid the temptation to re-open the conversation. A clear termination of the debrief takes the candidate out of the spotlight and allows the group to move on.

Summary and learning

Debrief is one of the most valuable aspects of teaching and learning, especially after simulations.

An effective debrief as a learning conversation is one where the facilitator listens to understand, and encourages the group to share their perspectives to help solve any puzzles that emerge.

Facilitators are encouraged to share their own perspective, describing what they have observed or heard, rather than asking leading questions.

Be honest, helpful and concrete in your feedback, engaging in an informative and relevant dialogue with the learners.

It's not what you tell them that counts, it's what they learn.

CHAPTER 9

Assessing

Introduction

Assessment is an essential element of the teaching and learning process for both candidates and instructors. Therefore getting assessment right is a key aim for instructors, and this chapter will give some essential underpinning theory and explore how to make assessments as reliable as possible.

Learning outcomes

This chapter will enable you to:

- Explain the purpose of assessment
- Describe different assessment types
- Explain the key principles behind assessments used on life support courses

Pocket Guide to Teaching for Clinical Instructors, Fourth Edition.
Edited by Kate Denning, Kevin Mackie and Alan Charters, Andrew Lockey.
© 2025 John Wiley & Sons Ltd. Published 2025 by John Wiley & Sons Ltd.

The purpose of assessment

Assessment plays a key role in education and has a number of discrete functions. It can be used to:

- Quantify or measure candidate achievement
- Support learning as part of an iterative process
- Focus and motivate learners
- Measure the effectiveness of teaching and learning
- Provide evidence to inform feedback for the learner and for the instructor
- Predict, to a degree, candidate performance when in work-based situations
- Reassure key stakeholders (including the wider public) about standards

On life support courses, the curriculum is made up of: the contents of the manual, which is knowledge-based; associated online learning, which serves as a bridge between the manual and the face to face element; and the application of that knowledge in the complex world of practical experience. It is this curriculum that is being assessed through a number of different formats, namely: multiple choice questionnaires (MCQs); skills and simulation assessment in both summative and formative formats; case-based discussions; and objective structured clinical exams (OSCEs).

Theoretical assessments of knowledge, whether they are embedded in online learning or take place on courses, have predetermined and consistent right/wrong answers. They are hard to write well, but that is not the concern of this chapter as instructors are not usually involved in writing them. The majority of the provider course assessment takes place at the face to face element of courses and this chapter will focus on the nuances of assessment and give some thoughts on ways in which instructors can carry out fair assessments to the best of their abilities.

The purpose of assessment is to measure the candidates' progress towards autonomy, as in Miller's pyramid and illustrated in Figure 9.1 (Miller, 1990). Within courses it is

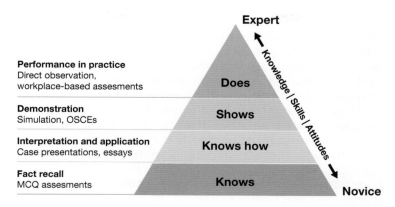

Figure 9.1 Miller's pyramid

possible to assess 'knows', 'knows how' and 'shows'. Attempts are made to assess 'does', but this is an ongoing process and ideally happens over a long period of time to mitigate against the forgetting curve.

Types of assessment

Traditionally, assessments have been described as formative (with an educational purpose) or summative (with an evaluative purpose). Formative assessment often occurs during a period of teaching or at strategic moments in a learner's journey and provides feedback that helps the learner make improvements. Summative assessment takes place at the end of a period of learning and does not have an ongoing educational role but provides a clear marker of a learner's skills and knowledge at that moment in time.

A useful analogy might be a chef preparing mushroom soup. They taste it and adjust ingredients/seasoning before serving. This mirrors formative assessment where frequent checking and good feedback lead to improvements. When they present the soup to the customer, a summative assessment of the final product takes place: at this point no further improvements can occur.

Assessment can also be seen as formal and informal. Whilst formal assessment is clearly signposted, the informal version takes place throughout any teaching session in which learners are active participants. Whenever facilitators make judgements about candidates, and this may be without necessarily realising that they are doing so, they are engaging in informal assessment and any decisions about whether the candidate has met the standards or not must be clearly communicated to them, even though the assessment is informal. This may be categorised as *'assessment **for** learning'* whereas summative assessment is *'assessment **of** learning'* (Westwood and Griffin, 2013).

There are disadvantages to all types of assessment, and each type has some compromises embedded. Largely, the provider courses have either summative, continuous or outcomes-based assessments. Summative assessments, which gather a host of experience into one short, intense assessment held at the end of the learning experience may misrepresent the individual through performance nerves. In an exam setting, some people do better and some worse than they do in practice settings.

One of the disadvantages of continuous or outcomes-based assessment is that those on the receiving end may view them as high stake and therefore the relentlessness of being repeatedly assessed can, for some, take over and prevent them taking risks and trying out new patterns of behaviour. However, Schut et al. (2018) found that the more learners were exposed to serial low stakes assessments, the less anxious they felt about them and therefore the more authentically they were able to behave. Despite these disadvantages, assessment is an essential component of life support courses and can be a real motivation for learning.

Assessment principles

Assessments are designed with five principles in mind: validity, reliability, feasibility, specificity and fidelity.

Validity

Validity is concerned with the content of the assessment:

- Are the right things being assessed? Does the assessment mirror the curriculum rather than assess comprehension of additional knowledge?
- Is the assessment a fair test? Is the appropriate, functioning equipment provided, for instance in a simulation?
- Does success in the assessment predict good future performance?

In order for assessment to be an accurate predictor of future performance, it would ideally consist of multiple assessment methods by many judges on many occasions spread out over a period of time. The more authentic to clinical reality the assessment is, the higher the validity. It is much harder to see how the candidate might behave in their own clinical practice when the setting of a simulation requires too much fabrication. The ideal of multiple assessments is not possible on short courses, and probably would not be very popular with candidates: different courses take different approaches to answering this challenge. Some use final summative assessment, others prefer serial outcomes-based assessment and yet others employ continuous assessment with ongoing opportunities for remediation where standards are not met.

Reliability

Reliability is concerned with the accuracy of the assessment, and asks the following questions:

- Is the assessment passing and failing the right candidates? Borderline cases present us with challenges about our decision making. Decisions about other candidates are relatively straightforward
- Do different instructors agree with each other?
- Would the candidate obtain a similar result if re-tested with the same or different instructors?

Assessment is an innately human process, which we each approach through the lens of our own experiences. Unfortunately, discrepancies in marking are a common theme in the literature on assessment, and while no instructor plans to carry out an unreliable assessment or to be biased, it happens because most of our biases are unconscious. Candidates need to feel confident that decisions reached during assessments are consistent and fair. In order to help with this, four supporting features can be found on life support and allied course.

Supporting reliable assessment decisions

1. The more complex assessments on life support courses are carried out by two or more instructors who are encouraged to communicate with each other about their decisions. This is because experts respond to slightly different bits of data and rather than ignoring this, it can be used to enhance reliability.
2. New instructors are paired with experienced instructors in order to learn about the community of practice. Novice assessors are often more hawk-like than dove-like and pairing instructors up should allow for moderation of potential issues.
3. Calibration is a key factor that many groups of assessors go through before they begin a series of assessments, though it is not explicitly done on provider courses. Difficult or potentially unclear criteria are, however, discussed at the faculty meeting prior to assessments so that instructors are all following the same principles as far as possible.
4. Assessment of skills and simulations are accompanied by checklists of key treatment points that need to be met and well-documented.

There is some evidence (Wilkinson et al., 2003) that global ratings are more valid than checklists, despite fears about subjectivity, when *examiners are experienced*. Key here is that it is experienced assessors who work best with the subjective nature of assessing professionalism; it is important therefore that new instructors are mentored until they have more experience in this area. When we are struggling to make a decision about someone, further information made by more decision-makers will help us reach a point of saturation, a point at which nothing will be added by further testing (van der Vleuten and Schuwirth, 2005).

Feasibility

There is a balance to be struck between reliability and validity, and this is described as the feasibility of the assessment. Measured against practical issues such as time and available resources, how feasible is it to carry out a specific type of assessment? Some are far more resource heavy than others. An MCQ requires a lot of work prior to the assessment, including writing, checking and validating the questions, but the moment of delivery is straightforward and requires few human resources. Many people can engage in an MCQ with only one official present, or they can be delivered online as pre-learning with no invigilation. Simulation assessments on the other hand are very resource heavy, requiring a minimum of two assessors and possibly a number of extra people to role play team members.

Summative assessments are relatively easy to run, with a clear distinction being made between teaching and assessing. It is important not to get involved in prompting the team leader, although they can be encouraged to share their thinking. There is some evidence that this is worth emphasising for international medical graduates in order to alleviate cross-cultural misunderstandings.

Continuous assessment, which meets the dual functions of learning and assessing concurrently, is an even more complex skill to acquire. Instructors need to help candidates when additional teaching is necessary. But they then need to ask themselves about the level of assistance that they gave. Consider the point in the course (the arc of learning) and make a decision as to whether the candidate is at the appropriately safe level or has not achieved that level yet and requires additional practice. These decisions must be communicated to candidates as they make progress in their learning journey.

Specificity

Assessment needs to be designed to ensure that the curriculum has been absorbed by the learners. Different formats relate to different domains of learning. Figure 9.2 indicates those that are used on the range of advanced life support courses.

Format	Description	Best for
Multiple choice questionnaire	These usually use a stem followed by a number of plausible options	Knowledge and understanding
Interactive online questions	There are different types of questions including single answer, multiple answers, ranking, prioritising and matching	Retrieval practice which is very useful for personal learning
Short answer questions	Short answer questions, often built into the pre-course learning	Bridging the gap between knowledge and application, prior to simulation practice
Skills test	Independent performance of a specific skill	Motor skills Sequences of actions
Simulation test	Enacting the role of team leader in a scenario	Application of algorithms The ability to lead on managing a seriously ill/injured/arrested patient Team work Professionalism An ABCDE assessment
Case-based discussions	Clinical cases Table top discussions	Planning and preparation Synthesis of knowledge
Objective structured clinical examination	A circuit of discrete stations	Multiple assessments of different but complementary knowledge

Figure 9.2 Forms of assessment

A multiple choice questionnaire, for example, is only useful in a specific context and for particular content; it is not good per se and in life support courses has mostly been removed from in-course assessment. In fact, none of these assessment methods gives a global picture. In order to gain an overall impression of a candidate's competency, courses should include more than one form of assessment.

Fidelity

Fidelity is about closeness to reality: authentic assessments are more informative and reliable than ones that are far removed from the environs to which the candidates will be returning after the course. It has been shown that authentic assessment, which echoes the real world situation as closely as possible, is a better predictor of performance, and more useful to the learners, than an assessment which does not mirror or is too far removed from practice.

Communicating assessment decisions

Summative assessment usually involves giving a 'result' indicating success or failure in meeting required outcomes. With continuous or outcomes-based assessment the communication of success, failure or progress must be made clear to candidates throughout the course and also during the debrief process. This sends a clear message of their level of performance at any given moment. Regardless of the type of assessment, it is important that candidates are aware of the benchmarks (e.g. what does a safe ABCDE assessment look like?) and can learn to calibrate themselves, often by getting full group input into learning conversations. Continuously assessed candidates should be given an opportunity to rectify areas in which they were not successful. The way this is done varies across different courses.

A teaching structure: practicalities of assessment

Whether assessment is formative, summative, outcomes-based or continuous, instructors have an obligation to know what is being assessed and how it is recorded. The following elements are applicable to all forms of practical assessment.

Prepare

Instructors need to know the assessment criteria themselves and should ensure that candidates also know the parameters. The instructors may have specific scenario details, but candidates must know the broad outlines on which they are being assessed. Equipment must be set up in advance so that the candidate can easily navigate the technical intricacies of assessment.

Open

Candidates need to be informed that an assessment is taking place. This is often obvious, but if formative or continuous assessment is taking place this should also be made clear. Roles of all participants should be established before the session begins. It can help candidates if an explanation of the practicalities of the assessment is given. For example, if the candidate will be asked to leave the room while the instructors hold a brief discussion, then let the candidates know that this will happen. Any time constraints should also be made clear so that abrupt termination is not seen as failure.

Facilitate

Give the candidate the information they need to proceed with the assessment, and offer timely clinical information if the equipment does not provide it directly. It is important to avoid prompting candidates, which might give them an unfair advantage, but you may question their thought processes or ask direct questions if needed. Clinical 'triggers' need to be given in a timely fashion, especially if the equipment is low fidelity. You may have to repeat triggers that are not immediately obvious; this is not prompting but will allow the assessment to flow naturally, enhancing fidelity.

Facilitating a simulation that combines teaching and assessment requires a less rigid approach because there has to be a balance between letting the session flow naturally and correcting any mistakes as they happen. Embedded faculty helpers can increase realism from within the simulation by comments such as '*The child is struggling more with their breathing than they were*', thus making it more likely that candidates will respond accurately to what is unfolding. Embedded helpers need, however, to give the candidates thinking time, so sometimes have to hold themselves back from intervening too quickly. As was stated earlier, if a candidate needs prompting in the continuous assessment setting then they should be. We need to be sure that candidates learn but also be reassured that they are safe. Discussion between instructors is important to ascertain whether a candidate was operating independently or was being coached through the scenario.

Close

You may need to confer with fellow instructors before reaching an assessment decision. In some situations, candidates are asked to leave the room whilst this interaction takes place, but with continuous or outcomes-based assessment it might be appropriate for the instructors to remove themselves from the scenario in order to reach a decision. Assessment decisions should be given clearly and succinctly. If the candidate has met the required outcomes, tell them so: if they have not, explain why and suggest how they may rectify any deficiencies. With continuous or outcomes-based assessment you will debrief the candidate with a learning conversation so that regardless of the outcome, learning will continue to happen.

Summary and learning

A variety of assessment techniques tests differing domains of learning.

Assessments need to be valid, reliable, feasible, specific and have fidelity.

Assessment decisions, whether formative or summative, must be clearly communicated to candidates.

Structure assessment around the 'Prepare, Open, Facilitate, Close' model.

CHAPTER **10**

Lectures and presentations

Introduction

The lecture is a relatively low-risk educational tool that enables a message to be reliably conveyed to a large group. At its best, the lecture is a means of transmitting knowledge in a standardised format. At its worst, it is based on a culture of silence, with lectures traditionally being seen and experienced as passively delivered events. With little planning or audience engagement a lecture can become a process by which the notes of the lecturer become the notes of the learner without passing through the mind of either. As has been shown in Chapter 1, there is a considerable body of evidence showing that, if adult learners are to benefit from an educational event, active learning is required. This chapter will explore ways in which a lecture can be interactive, providing a more powerful experience for both teacher and learners. Increasingly we are employing online lectures and webinars, this will also be touched upon in this chapter.

Pocket Guide to Teaching for Clinical Instructors, Fourth Edition.
Edited by Kate Denning, Kevin Mackie and Alan Charters, Andrew Lockey.
© 2025 John Wiley & Sons Ltd. Published 2025 by John Wiley & Sons Ltd.

> ## Learning outcomes
>
> This chapter will enable you to:
> - Explain the value and limitations of the lecture
> - Plan an engaging and interactive lecture
> - Formulate different types of questions

Benefits and challenges of lectures

Disseminating information

The lecture enables specific messages to be conveyed to a group of learners. The advent of webinars has meant that lectures can be watched by millions of viewers simultaneously, either live or pre-recorded. More commonly, for example in life support courses, groups are likely to be relatively small (12–30 people). Nevertheless, it is an opportunity to give a particular message to all the learners at the same time and to repeat exactly the same message to other groups. This does not necessarily mean that the same message has been *received* by all individuals in the room, since they interpret the content through the lens of their individual experiences and understanding of the topic.

Reducing ambiguity

Lectures rarely break new ground, they are much more likely to provide the opportunity to clarify information learned in other contexts – for example reading a text or watching a demonstration. Questions, in both directions, will enhance this process.

Stimulating learner interest

When you ask people to recall the best lecture they have ever heard, they are more likely to comment on the personal style, charisma and entertainment value of the lecturer than on its actual content. What lecturers are doing in these cases is motivating their learners, albeit subtly, to go away and do some reading and thinking about the subject.

Introducing content

Lectures can lay the foundations for more detailed study by signposting learners in particular directions.

Limitations

Lectures do have limitations, including the fact that skills cannot be taught, and that it is difficult to present complex and/or abstract ideas in a comprehensible manner. However, the main disadvantage is one of learner attention span, which varies considerably among learners but is probably between 10 and 30 minutes. The effectiveness of lectures depends on a variety of factors, particularly levels of engagement.

A teaching structure: delivering a lecture

As described in Chapter 3, a structure (Prepare, Open, Facilitate, Close) can be applied to any teaching session. Lectures are no exception.

Prepare

Take care to check the venue before you give your lecture, arriving in plenty of time before you are due to speak.

- *Check the layout:* The room may already be set up for a lecture (i.e. rows of chairs facing a screen) but a horseshoe may be more appropriate for a smaller group.
- *Test the projection facilities:* In most cases, you will find a computer and data projector readily available, but make sure you are familiar with the computer, where to put your flash drive, and whether there is a remote control. For peace of mind, have a back-up for your presentation. One way of doing this is to email your presentation to yourself and/or the local organiser, or have it available on cloud-based storage.
- *Adjust temperature and lighting:* If the room has been occupied for some time, open windows or run the air conditioning; make sure that your slides are visible with lights on or slightly dimmed (beware of making the room too dark, providing a potentially sleep-inducing setting).

- **Check for a clock:** If there is not one visible, remind yourself to use your watch. Contrary to opinion, it is not distracting for a lecturer to keep an eye on the time.

When teaching online the specific preparation you need to make prior to the teaching event in many ways mirrors your preparation for teaching face to face.

- **Check your own layout:** Try to set your camera up so that the lighting is on you, and your face and shoulders fill the screen. It is a little more flattering if you are looking slightly upwards, and worth avoiding a cluttered background. Ask colleagues whether your sound is working well; you may even need to ask people in the same building as you to avoid streaming while you are lecturing online, particularly if you need to share video content.
- **Ensure familiarity with platform:** Test the platform for sharing content and ensure you can still see at least some of the participants. It may be helpful to nominate someone to monitor the people and the chat for you: this will ensure a better experience for the group. Consider the use of virtual breakout rooms for discussions; these usually need to be set up before the event, or by someone other than the lecturer.
- **Cameras:** Decide whether or not participants in a remote lecture should have their cameras on. In a life support course, where attendance at all elements is compulsory, candidates must be visible for at least part of the remote lecture.
- **Timing:** Keep an eye on time during your session.

Open

Your slides should include learning outcomes, showing what you expect the group to know by the end of the session. The first minute or so of your lecture is your opportunity to claim credibility, by virtue of who you are and what you do. The learners will already have made an assessment based on your appearance, but they need to be reassured that you are qualified to be introducing the topic to them.

Consider the kind of atmosphere you hope to create. You probably want the group of learners to engage with you, and to share their knowledge when given the opportunity, but you may prefer it if they wait for a signal from you before talking. You may need to exercise some control to avoid people talking over each other or going off at a tangent. Humour is an under-valued resource that has the effect of relaxing the group. If you feel able to introduce some gentle laughter, and this is a much broader remit than telling jokes with great comic timing, then you will reap the benefits as the group warm to you. However, it is probably advisable that you use humour only if it comes naturally, and even then use it sparingly and appropriately.

Facilitate

At this stage cover the content and the substance of the learning outcomes you introduced at the beginning of the lecture. In most cases, you will be working from pre-prepared slide sets that have an approved content. In other cases, you will be presenting your own slides. Whatever the situation, much of the experience for the learners will be in *how* you present your information, rather than the information itself. In fact, some experts argue that only 7% of communication is about the words you speak, as Figure 10.1 suggests. This raises some important issues when considering the components of what makes a successful presentation.

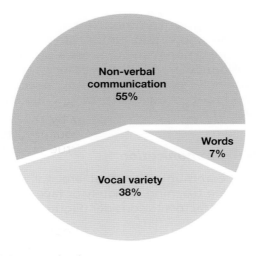

Figure 10.1 Communication

Vocal variety

Vocal variety or verbal style refers to:

- Voice
- Emphasis
- Pace
- Enthusiasm

You might think that there is nothing you can do about your voice, but that is not entirely the case. Pitch and projection are two elements that will help you to be heard. Certain sections of the content may need emphasis – you will develop a personal style as to how this can be achieved. Strategies range from speaking a little louder than normal, slowing down and repetition, modulating your voice or simply telling the learners to make note of what you are about to say. The pace at which you speak is important even when you are not expecting your group to take notes. Slightly slower than normal conversation gives your learners time to reflect and, for anyone listening in a second language, it gives a chance for deeper comprehension. Enthusiasm is contagious, as unfortunately is its opposite. Generally, you should communicate keenness for your subject by speaking with a degree of animation. Overenthusiasm, however, may distract leaners from the content of your lecture.

Verbal or physical mannerisms can become a distraction – learners might focus on how many times you use a word, phrase or on some physical trait rather than absorbing what you are saying. Common verbal mannerisms are 'OK', 'so...', 'you know' and 'umm'. Linguists call these 'hesitation phenomena', and they are a product of habit, lack of confidence or working memory capacity. More often than not, speakers are not aware of their mannerisms so it is advisable to get feedback from colleagues.

Non-verbal communication

Elements of communication that are not verbal apply whether you are teaching remotely or face to face. There are a number of factors to consider (Figure 10.2).

Gesture	Use natural gestures
Posture	Look relaxed
Position	Both sides of the room at different times, avoiding the projector beam
Proximity	Close enough without invading personal space
Movement	Move naturally and purposefully (i.e. to get closer to someone who is asking or answering a question)
Eye contact	Sweep the room at eye level, taking in everyone
Facial expression	Look interested, smile

Figure 10.2 Non-verbal communication

Words

The words you speak are clearly important and even when you are using course slides you are in control of what you say. It is not advisable to read off the slides themselves or memorise a script because you are less likely to engage the learners and also less likely to notice their response if they misunderstand or disengage. You may also sound a little stilted. In essence, use the slides as prompts to enable a more natural and confident delivery. If you feel the need for security, however, you might want to put bullet points or keywords on small index cards. In general, however, the slides should be enough to remind you of what you want to say.

Interaction

Some attention has to be paid to interaction within your lecture, however short it is. As we have already discussed, there are serious limitations on what you can achieve and how long you can maintain everyone's attention by talking *at* the group. There is a balance to be met between transmission of knowledge and receiving the group's thoughts. Absorbing lectures are those that create opportunities to allow the learners to explore and engage with the ideas in conversation with other learners and with you as a facilitator. This can broadly be done by asking questions and by setting interactive tasks (Table 10.1).

Setting interactive tasks

Table 10.1 Interactions within the lecture	
Type of interaction	**Example**
Opportunities for individual reflection	How does this concept fit in with your previous experience? How might you integrate this new approach in your practice?
Pairs and small group discussion, e.g. problem-solving, sharing information or experiences	Talk to your neighbour about the last time you met a similar scenario. What might have improved the outcome?
Prioritising, sequencing, sorting	Have a go at triaging these four patients

In each of the examples your best response is to take contributions from enough people to show that you are interested in what they have to say without completely going over all the ground again, which may seem like a waste of time to the learners. Whether working remotely or face to face, try not to focus on any one group, but draw contributions from different groups.

In a face to face setting, people telegraph the desire to speak in a number of ways, leaning forward, slightly raising their hand, fidgeting in their seat, etc. Online some people diligently use the 'hands up' function, others join in spontaneously. When lecturing remotely it can be useful to have a list of the names of the candidates so that you can keep a record of who has contributed and make sure to include the more reticent ones. The internet is now more familiar to most of us, but fluent online tutoring still takes some practice.

Asking questions

Questions are an important way of achieving dialogue and interactivity. Bloom et al. (1956) describe six levels in the cognitive domain, building in complexity as you move up the diagram. They require different ways of asking questions in order to achieve the necessary outcome (Figure 10.3).

Evaluation: Making comparisons, for example '*What are the benefits and drawbacks of measuring and treating altered pH levels in emergency situations?*'

Synthesis: Putting knowledge of one subject together with that of another, for example '*How would we approach the treatment of a patient with a pH of 7.2?*'

Analysis: Checking the significance, for example '*What implications does a blood pH of 7.2 have on our approach to treatment?*'

Application: Exploring the relevance, for example '*In what situations would we need to ascertain the patient's pH?*'

Comprehension: Checking understanding, for example '*What does pH tell us about the acid-base status of a patient?*'

Knowledge: Seeking factual information, for example '*What is the normal pH?*'

Figure 10.3 Different ways of asking questions

Some of these questions lend themselves more readily to workshops than to the lecture theatre but they all enhance learner buy-in and enjoyability.

Regardless of the cognitive level of questions you use, you can ask questions in a number of ways:

- **Questions to random, named individuals:** These are intended to keep learners on their toes, but can be intimidating. People placed under considerable pressure by this approach may forget things that they would reasonably be expected to know.
- **Questions along a row:** Asking ten people in turn to name ten known facts has a number of negative effects: the first person has many options open to them, the second person, one fewer and so on. By the time you get to the eighth person, there are only three left and pressure along the row will almost certainly guarantee that they will not be able to contribute. In the meantime, learners in the first few positions can take a break and possibly lose concentration.
- **Pose, pause, pounce:** This is a common strategy, encouraging all the learners to think of a possible answer before someone (who may look as if they know) is invited to respond. But it is not very popular with those learners who find it threatening.
- **Questions to the group as a whole:** This gives everyone the opportunity to demonstrate their knowledge and insight. If the question has been phrased appropriately and at the right level, someone will usually be able to answer it.
- **Questions to part of the group:** This is a subset of the above and can be useful when, for example, the same person keeps answering questions, or nobody answers. By asking, '*Anyone in the middle row*' or '*This side of the room*' the focus is narrowed down, making people more likely to (feel pressure to) respond.
- **Questions from the group:** Your questions to the group may also generate questions *from* the group, which may reveal a misunderstanding or omission from your lecture and give you an opportunity to correct it in your immediate answer and/or your summary.

Whatever the strategy, you need to respond in certain ways, assuming for the moment that the answer is correct.

Responding to questions

- Acknowledge it
- Repeat or paraphrase the answer (some people talk very quietly and others may not hear them)
- Expand on the response (particularly if it is partial)
- Ask supplementary question(s)
- Relate it to other parts of your lecture (if relevant)

If not relevant, politely bring the focus back to the course content; the likelihood is that respondents will answer correctly. However, you do need to be prepared for two phenomena: the wrong answer and complete silence. Both can be important but various strategies are used to deal with them. Consider these examples.

Example

Instructor: *'Does anyone know the correct dose of amiodarone administered after the 3rd shock?'*

Candidate: *'1 mg'*

Instructor: *'I think you are probably thinking of adrenaline, the right answer is 300 mg. It's fine though to look up doses if you are in the least bit unsure'*

In this example, the instructor has corrected a factual error without saying 'No that was wrong'. Fear of getting the answer wrong is one of the factors that prevents us from answering questions. Always acknowledge a contribution even if it is wrong. As you can see from the example above, the instructor acknowledges the answer and confirms that 1 mg was the right answer to a different question before giving the correct information, so that all of the candidates know the correct answer and do not leave confused or misinformed.

Example

Instructor: '*OK. Who can tell me what the energy presence, essential for contraction and relaxation of muscle fibres, within cardiac muscles is?*'

Candidate/s: [Silence]

Instructor (after a suitable pause): '*The answer is ATP, can anyone tell me what ATP stands for?*'

Candidate: '*Adenosine triphosphate*'

Instructor: '*That's right, what about how it works?*'

Candidate: '*Doesn't it allow the muscles to re-contract?*'

Instructor: '*Yes, that's the basic principle. What you need to know for this course is that without ATP, cardiac muscles would remain in their contracted state, rather than their relaxed state*'

This example uses an approach where a complex question is followed by simpler questions. Candidates may know the answer, but this technique allows them a more concrete basis for their response. Breaking the question down simplifies it and makes it relevant to the course learning outcomes. We do not expect our learners to be 'walking textbooks', but certain bits of knowledge are important for comprehension and application.

Obviously, there should be variations on these themes, using your own language, but you should always aim to be supportive rather than critical or sarcastic. Whatever strategies you adopt, they should lead to interactions that enable the learners to share, with you and everyone else, a more certain understanding of the subject.

Close

At the end of your lecture or presentation be sure to leave enough time to ask for questions and respond to them, before summarising and closing the session.

Asking for questions (and waiting for long enough for them to be voiced) gives learners the opportunity to resolve any uncertainties they may have. In general, it is safe to treat these as genuine requests for information and to answer them succinctly. On occasion, this might include owning up to not knowing the answer, in which case never guess at or invent an answer. Your credibility will not be diminished by consulting faculty colleagues or saying that you will find the right answer and let people know, or by asking them to re-phrase the question.

The occasional individual may ask a question such as '*I read in a recent edition of the Annals of Emergency Medicine that...*'. This learner may well be trying to impress you but is probably also keen to demonstrate that they are knowledgeable and well read. However this makes you feel, it is vital, as always, that your response does not undermine the candidate.

The summary is your opportunity to give candidates a 'take-home message': it should relate directly to the learning outcomes as detailed in your opening of the course. Once more, it should be succinct and not revisit the whole content of your lecture. The summary comes after questions – so that the lecture does not run over time ('*I can accept one more question before I summarise*') and learners leave with your take-home message fresh in their minds.

Termination is important because it avoids the situation in which the learners are not sure what is going to happen next. Say something like '*Right, wait here as Professor Angstrom is going to talk to you about a new way of thinking about the control of type 1 diabetes*' or '*Thanks for your attention, and now it's time for coffee. Please be back by 11.15*'. This is preferable to the candidates sitting uncertainly while the lecturer shuffles papers or recovers a data stick.

Summary and learning

A lecture is an opportunity to give many learners the same message.

Lectures are not always giving 'new' information but may remind people of what they have come across in other contexts.

Lectures are not good for delivering complex knowledge or practical skills, but they do have a distinct and recognisable place in learning.

Use techniques such as questioning to engage learners and hopefully improve their knowledge and understanding.

CHAPTER 11

Blended learning

Introduction

In this book we have mainly considered face to face learning environments, though we have mentioned online learning as being a common factor in most life support courses, especially pre-course study. Blended learning uses various methods, combining face to face interactions with online activities, which will suit different learning styles and preferences. Here, we explore these areas and see how they apply in the context of life support courses.

Learning outcomes

This chapter will enable you to:

- Describe and support the development of the blended learning experience from the perspective of the candidate
- Define where blended learning is currently used

Pocket Guide to Teaching for Clinical Instructors, Fourth Edition.
Edited by Kate Denning, Kevin Mackie and Alan Charters, Andrew Lockey.
© 2025 John Wiley & Sons Ltd. Published 2025 by John Wiley & Sons Ltd.

Blended learning in the context of life support courses

Most life support courses use blended learning with a combination of a virtual learning environment (VLE) and a face to face course. It is part of the instructor's role to provide a seamless link between the two by knowing the format and content of the pre-course learning.

Digital elements used in courses include:

- Virtual learning environments
- e-manuals
- Discussion boards
- Online teaching: synchronous
- Online teaching: asynchronous

In contrast to pure online learning, blended learning offers a mixture of remote and face to face delivery, empowering candidates to work at their own speed and at a time and place convenient to them, thus enabling self-direction. Blended learning is not simply delivering elements of face to face learning online, although the content is informed by the learning outcomes for the course. From design to delivery, a blended learning approach should exploit the benefits of all the varying elements.

Most health education organisations now use blended learning as part of a planned digital strategy. Developing digital literacy skills is essential to contemporary teaching and learning, and may enhance employability.

Blended learning allows candidate to choose how and when they access certain aspects of the course. This includes the use of mobile devices.

Potential benefits

Over the past decade or so, we have seen improved understanding of technology and its contribution to creating meaningful learning opportunities. Technological advantages, such as interactivity and multi-media platforms, have been exploited to create some innovative, engaging and enjoyable learning resources.

Highly publicised workforce pressures in healthcare make it difficult for both learners and instructors to be released from work to attend long periods of study. The international trend for educational courses has been to reduce face to face time and adopt a blended learning approach. Recent changes to ways of working, such as increased awareness of online communication platforms, have pushed the boundaries of 'what' and 'how' online content is delivered. This is particularly evident in 'live' or synchronous elements where facilitators are present online at the same time as learners. This upsurge in the use of online platforms means that teachers and learners are now much more familiar with the technology and elements formerly regarded as 'needing to be delivered face to face' (e.g. exams). These are now routinely managed online. Online learning as part of a blended approach has significant benefits for the learner, the faculty, and their environment, which can include:

- It is easier to negotiate time to study if you have flexible access and you do not have to be in a specific place (this works well for shift workers, who generally prefer the blended approach)
- Reduced need for travel (lowers carbon footprint and reduces time away from work or home) and is more cost efficient
- Instructors' ability to control the dynamics, creating personal pathways for learners
- Increased opportunity to track engagement and trigger support
- The fact that blended learning approaches may increase comprehension in the face to face elements
- Ability to increase learner numbers
- More efficient use of instructor time
- Consistency of theoretical messaging not reliant on human communication

Potential limitations

- Distractions in the chosen learning environment, such as other people, music or television
- Unreliable internet access
- A candidate's belief that they retain information more easily from face to face learning than from online content

Considerations in the development of blended learning

The blended learning experience should be planned holistically, giving consideration to all learning styles and preferences and 'how' you want the learners to interact. Quinn (2012) identified four ways to interact with course materials, which are summarised in Figure 11.1.

Content: Considers the benefits of sharing content with the learners so they can access, view or store.

Compute: Concerns learners using their device to compute. For example, they might enter some clinical values or a drug calculation, using the online learning to compute the result. We see this in online drug calculators and poison-specific advice sites

Capture: Is about the learner capturing and producing content for themselves, rather than accessing it. They may be tasked with capturing videos of themselves practising a skill or delivering a lecture, useful where the learning outcome is to 'demonstrate'.

Communicate: Sharing data, text, or any type of multi-media to communicate with other learners and/or a facilitator. This can happen in synchronous interaction, where everyone is online at the same time, using real-time communication; or asynchronous interaction, such as in a discussion board or chat that functions offline.

Figure 11.1 Four ways to interact with course content

Varying the style and content of teaching resources will engage the majority of learners (Figure 11.2).

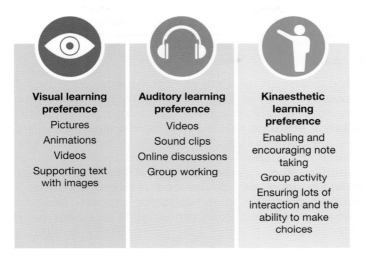

Figure 11.2 Learning preferences

Examples of the range of activities that can be incorporated into digital teaching resources are:

- Reading text
- Links to relevant resources and websites
- Different question types to encourage learners to engage in retrieval practice
- Case studies to work through, with open answer text boxes to aid application of earlier knowledge
- Game-like activities such as matching, filling in blanks, 'moving' pieces of equipment or choosing the most appropriate action
- Enhanced reality-simulated experiences
- Audio or video resources to watch
- Images to enhance the look of the content
- Branching scenarios with different pathways depending on decisions made
- Discussion groups

Other considerations include the need to offer reflective learning prompts in the form of journal-type entries which can be saved and collated, and creating opportunities for analysis of concepts, ideas and content in a systematic way. Some learners need to understand the whole picture, rather than having it built up in smaller components, such as summaries, abstracts and overviews. Balancing all of these different needs can be a challenge when designing online learning.

Application in life support courses

Prepare

Some courses may use a pre-course discussion board to support learners in their preparations. Discussion boards aim to mitigate psychological and communicational distance, ensuring that learners have a sense of the group they are learning with and feel able to 'talk' to the group. Asking questions in these forums encourages peer responses and a feeling of shared learning. Instructors should engage with discussions in a timely manner and respond positively to requests for support, or redirect learners to support each other if this does not happen spontaneously.

Literature suggests that there are two types of active learner on a discussion board; the 'lurkers' and the 'posters', but there are also inactive learners or 'non-users'. The definitions of 'posters' and 'non-users' are self-explanatory, but the notion of the educational benefit of 'lurkers' is interesting and something worth considering. In internet culture, lurking has been frowned upon, active participation being preferred. Taking active part is still encouraged, but educational research suggests that 'lurking' can be highly beneficial and, for many learners, just as important as the active participation we see from 'posters'. For the reflective learner, reading the posts and reflecting upon their content has high educational value.

Many of our courses offer pre-course learning by accessing online content through a learning management system (LMS) or VLE. We check that candidates have completed the mandatory online learning, but we do not delve into the length of time each individual spends on each section, even though this information is available to us. Many adults are 'self-directed' and have a preference for varying materials and preparatory techniques. Online learning modules can be either mandatory or optional, allowing candidates to tailor their learning whilst also meeting the essential outcomes set by the course.

Pre-course learning on life support courses uses a mixture of pedagogical theories and ensures that a range of activities are offered to meet the needs of differing learning styles or preferences, and to add variety.

When preparing for online delivery, consider whether your session is going to be live or pre-recorded, and how your environment will affect the sound quality. Some research suggests that friendly background sound marks the instructor as human and relatable, but distracting or loud background noise will affect learning; so consider your chosen location and how you may prevent interruptions to both your delivery and your concentration. If you will be visible on screen, try to use plain, obstacle-free or blurred backgrounds that do not distract other participants. Greenscreen image backgrounds can be used, though be sure to check and test that they work fully; they will create a distraction if they are unstable.

If using video or other media (either embedded or streaming), test it beforehand and have a back-up plan in case of problems. Common causes of error include linking to the internet from a location with poor Wi-Fi connection and/or the presence of a firewall that does not permit access. Bandwidth of internet connections can be unreliable so it is a good idea to check beforehand.

Open

When delivering online content, spend a few moments at the start setting expectations. This may include switching off email notifications, promoting the use of headphones where appropriate and providing clarity on how you wish candidates to engage with the session: for example, using the raised hand technique or posting in the 'chat' panel. Consider the use of a briefed co-instructor for 'chat' management rather than trying to deliver a lecture or facilitate a discussion while also keeping watch on the 'chat'. Confirm whether computer cameras are to be switched on or off; this is a debatable topic, some organisations having strict rules, others allowing choice. Ensure this is discussed in advance so that everyone receives the same message. From an instructor's perspective, it can be incredibly difficult to lecture to a virtual space with nobody in sight; however, it can be equally distracting with the cameras on. Reading facial expressions can also be harder online than in the classroom.

Facilitate

The temptation to 'read along' the slides can be more prevalent in an online session. Ensure your dialogue complements the slides. Text on a screen can be difficult to read, so consider the use of images to stimulate thought.

Online poll software such as Slido®, Doodle® or Mentimeter® can help with engagement and allow you to manage multiple inputs. Most of the basic versions of these platforms or 'apps' are free to use and create graphics based on responses that you can then show on-screen and discuss. Again, it is advisable to have a second person to support you in managing the data, to prevent your becoming distracted.

If you are sharing your screen, make sure that the device settings are enabled for sound and for moving forward to the next slide or content. It is a good idea to have any content opened but minimised on your desktop to allow quick selection.

Most candidates, being familiar with the problems of technology, will accept the occasional delay, but if you appear completely out of your depth your credibility will be affected and learners may disengage.

Instructors who are used to receiving immediate feedback in a classroom may find it challenging when their humorous asides are met with a wall of silence. You just have to carry on and imagine the 'laugh' in your head. In order to sound more genuine, you should try to speak in your normal manner.

Close

Ideally, you should appear to speak to each learner individually to enable them to ask questions. If you have been sharing your screen, stop sharing and (if possible) check each participant separately for visual clues as to whether they are trying to formulate a question or are seeking clarity. You can ask them to display reactive emojis (thumbs up, raised hand) to help you deal with specific questions, or you might find the chat function useful, although it is not easy to read and speak at the same time. This is where the moderator or helper can assist by filtering and vocalising candidates' questions. Closing is fairly straightforward: you formulate your summary and final remarks and then close the session.

Summary and learning

Blended learning is increasingly being used in most life support courses.

Face-to-face content cannot simply be transferred online.

Learners should not be left unsupported during online learning.

Exploiting technology to enhance learning in a well-planned and organised way is valued by learners.

CHAPTER 12

Non-technical skills

Introduction

Non-technical skills (NTS) comprise individual and team cognitive or social attributes that support technical skills, especially when performing complex tasks. An awareness of NTS is particularly important for practitioners engaged in high-stress situations. As an instructor, therefore, you must consider NTS in the same light as the technical knowledge exhibited by candidates on courses.

Learning outcomes

This chapter will enable you to:

- Define the terms 'human factors' and 'non-technical skills'
- Describe team behaviours relevant to clinical team communication:
  - read-back
  - directed communication
  - closed loop communication
- Choose educational techniques to help train people in non-technical skills

---

Pocket Guide to Teaching for Clinical Instructors, Fourth Edition.
Edited by Kate Denning, Kevin Mackie and Alan Charters, Andrew Lockey.
© 2025 John Wiley & Sons Ltd. Published 2025 by John Wiley & Sons Ltd.

What are human factors and non-technical skills?

Human factors (HF) is the term used to describe the relationship between humans (cognitive), the tools and equipment they use (physical), and the environment in which they work (organisational) (Figure 12.1).

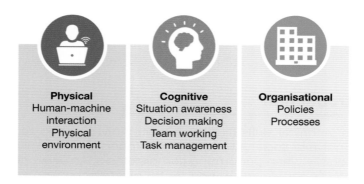

Physical
Human-machine interaction
Physical environment

Cognitive
Situation awareness
Decision making
Team working
Task management

Organisational
Policies
Processes

Figure 12.1 Human factors

Non-technical skills (NTS) are associated with social, cognitive and personal skills that can enhance the way that technical know-how, tasks and procedures are carried out. By developing these skills, people in safety-critical roles can learn how to deal with a range of different situations, to minimise error and to enhance patient safety.

So, NTS are the tools we use to minimise risk caused by a breakdown in HF within a team, and they broadly fit into the following categories:

- Leadership and teamwork
- Workload management
- Situation awareness
- Decision making
- Communication

Leadership and teamwork

Coordination of action with other team members is crucial, requiring the exchange of information and instructions. When issuing instructions, team leaders can make appropriate use of assertiveness. An important duty for the team leader is to understand the capabilities of each team member, and to support them when needed.

Workload management

Where possible, teams should gather in advance for planning and role allocation. This can be difficult when responding to an unexpected call, but it need not be a lengthy process. Prioritisation of tasks is crucial, especially in the early stages of a scenario where resources (particularly staff) may be limited. Good leaders know which resources are available, and how these may change as a situation evolves. Resources include obvious things like people or equipment, but also less tangible items such as support systems or guidelines.

Situation awareness

Situation awareness means understanding a scenario by gathering information, interpreting it and then using it to anticipate events. Note that situation awareness does not operate only at the level of individual team members: *'team situation awareness'* represents the understanding of the whole team. In a complex scenario it is unlikely that everyone on the team can maintain the same situation awareness at all times. Team members must therefore find appropriate moments to update colleagues who have missed some vital event.

Decision making

Decision making is a cyclical process, involving iden-tification of possible options before evaluating the risks and benefits of each. Depending on experience and circumstances, this evaluation might require time for conscious, systematic appraisal. Other choices might be made very quickly, and largely instinctively. Finally, the impact of decisions must be assessed, and plans updated accordingly.

Communication

Communication, as a NTS, refers to the ability to effectively convey and exchange information, ideas and emotions with others through various means such as speaking, writing, body language and active listening. It involves clarity, coherence, empathy and the capacity to tailor messages to the other person's needs and context, ensuring mutual understanding and fostering positive interpersonal relationships. Using people's names when allocating tasks and closing the communication loop are essential elements of communication in life support courses as will be explored later.

Why should we train people in non-technical skills?

You may well recall cases where resuscitation was unsuccessful but staff were able to accept a poor outcome knowing that everything possible was done. Conversely, it is possible for a team to leave a scenario feeling uneasy, even where the patient survived. How teams reflect on their performance is not based solely on patient outcome, but also on how efficiently care was delivered.

The need to train people in technical skills, such as safe defibrillation, requires little justification, but this has not always been the case for NTS. Previously NTS were not formally taught, so it was largely chance whether a team would demonstrate good skills or not. Formal training allows an opportunity for teams to develop these skills consciously and consistently.

Good NTS mean that teams work cohesively, and strong NTS performance is associated with the delivery of better care (Riem et al., 2012). This can be difficult in healthcare, where membership of clinical teams is often transitory. Clinicians often work with colleagues they have not previously met or have worked with only briefly. Training people to use standardised approaches like ABCDE, cognitive aids (resuscitation algorithms, for instance) or sharing information using handover tools are simple methods that can lend consistency as team membership changes.

Unlike technical skills, self-assessment of NTS is generally unreliable (Arora et al., 2011). There is, therefore, an important role for you as an instructor in facilitating reflection on NTS performance, especially during debriefing. This is a good time to involve the wider group of learners who are sometimes able to see things as observers that they cannot see when they themselves are 'performing'.

Human performance limitation

The value of HF lies in understanding how humans perform under pressure. Many skills, both technical and non-technical, are degraded by high levels of workload. This effect can be illustrated by the Yerkes–Dodson relationship, which describes how performance varies with workload (Figure 12.2). At very high operating tempo people become overloaded, and it is not surprising that they cannot give their best. Counter-intuitively, performance can also suffer at very low workload. This is largely because people become disengaged or bored, and so do not focus fully.

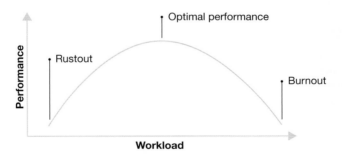

Figure 12.2 The Yerkes–Dodson relationship

The Yerkes–Dodson relationship highlights one reason why it is important that team leaders do not also perform clinical care tasks. There is a continuum between thinking and acting – the more one is done, the less room there is for the other. Practical tasks should therefore be delegated to ensure that the team leader does not become saturated.

You may recall being involved in performing chest compressions during a simulation on a life support course and being asked during debrief to give your thoughts on the management of the situation. Team members are often unable to give any feedback because they cannot focus on the task in hand and the bigger picture. As you observe candidates practising being a team leader you can encourage them to take responsibility for ensuring that team members have sufficient capacity to perform their roles, and balance tasks between colleagues. We can also encourage team members to recognise when they are absorbed, and to speak up when their situation awareness is needed.

Workload affects situation awareness through the ability to absorb and process information. The more task-focused someone becomes, the less likely they are to notice events around them. This is called a 'perceptual error', and can occur with visual, auditory or tactile stimuli. These phenomena explain why sometimes people appear to miss important cues from clinical monitors or seem to ignore colleagues. Vulnerability to these errors is universal, but people vastly overestimate their ability to notice critical events when under pressure. People may not therefore realise how important their team's contribution to situation awareness is.

Once information has been gathered it can be used to make choices. Four different ways of reaching decisions have been described (Figure 12.3): creative, analytical, rules-based or recognition-primed (Glavin, 2011).

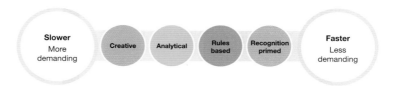

Figure 12.3 Decision making

Creative decisions are the most complex, made when a solution must be reasoned from first principles. Analytical decisions take somewhat less effort, and occur in situations where choices can be made from a defined list of options. Each must be evaluated to reach the optimal solution, which still takes some time. Rules-based decisions are straightforward to make provided the clinician recognises which rule applies, for example when determining if a rhythm is shockable or non-shockable. The least cognitively demanding decisions are recognition-primed. These are made instinctively and take almost no conscious effort.

Decision making is compromised by high workload, for example when less time is available to identify options. This can cause 'premature closure', when evaluation of options is stopped before all reasonable possibilities have been considered. Various cognitive biases might unduly weigh on the decision too, so sometimes slowing a team down to allow them to evaluate options properly can actually save time by improving efficiency.

Generally, the cognitive limitations described here are innate, so little can be done directly to reduce an individual's vulnerability. Instead, your role as an instructor is to focus on helping teams mitigate the risk. Good teamwork, through support and information sharing, may be one of the best means of maintaining overall performance.

Non-technical skills on life support courses

Traditionally, NTS were taught by the 'hidden curriculum' which represents all the things that people are taught without either the instructor being aware they are teaching or the learner being aware they are learning. These behaviours and skills are developed by informal observation of role models. Now that NTS have been better codified, it is possible to encourage specific reflection, offer guidance and suggest new techniques or methods with which to experiment.

Using these skills depends on interaction with others; they are difficult to learn from books or practise in a classroom. Small group work can be a useful way to encourage reflection, and to review successes or barriers, but practising NTS in depth requires a group performing a task together. On provider courses this most often happens during simulations.

A useful way to teach both situation awareness and decision making is to invite a prediction before starting an intervention. After a suitable period has passed, assess the decision's impact. In a clinical environment, this can be a powerful technique when assessing a new patient. Imagine performing an assessment on someone with hypoxia and an audible wheeze. You make a diagnosis of asthma, and start treatment with nebulisers. You make an explicit prediction that their wheeze will lessen and their oxygenation will improve. If your prediction comes true, it will reassure you that your diagnosis and initial management were correct. If, however, the prediction does not come true, it forces you to repeat your assessment. If the patient remains hypoxic despite improved wheezing, your treatment is appropriate but perhaps you need more of it. Alternatively, perhaps your diagnosis is not correct? Could you have missed an important piece of information, such as hyper-resonance indicating a pneumothorax? Forcing yourself to look for alternative diagnoses that might fit the symptoms and signs you have observed can make your situation awareness more reliable.

Encouraging colleagues to verbalise their interpretation of a situation (their 'mental model') can help the team by ensuring that everyone shares the same understanding. Also, inviting your candidate to offer a real-time commentary at key points can help you monitor their performance. This allows you to know best when and how to offer support.

When carrying out a decision, which might be either real or hypothetical, there is an opportunity for instructors to ask the candidate to describe all available resources. This can include the human resources they can draw on, the equipment they can access or the guidelines and systems that are applicable to their case. It is not necessarily natural to consider such things as resources, but activating systems such as major haemorrhage or cardiac arrest bring vital expertise and materials swiftly to the bedside.

Discussing these options openly can prompt reflection on less intuitive aspects of work.

Non-technical skills in simulation

Simulation is well placed for exploring NTS performance, particularly during situations where in reality there may be neither capacity nor psychological safety to fully reflect on performance. As explored in Chapter 6, meaningful NTS teaching opportunities need not require highly realistic manikins. Simulations offer many opportunities for observation of technical and non-technical skills.

Debriefing needs to be handled with good judgement because in many cases you will want to access the learners' internal processes. In order to explore decision making, for example, you might find it worthwhile to encourage the team leader to reflect on how and why they reached a decision; and for the rest of the group to reflect on how aware they were of the decision-making process. If you, or anyone in the group, would have made a different choice, this can be shared to provide the launching pad for a productive conversation about factors that affect the decisions we make.

Where available, video-assisted debriefing can be very powerful. Using video assistance takes training and experience, but offers the ability to enhance debrief with playback of selected recordings. This can be particularly valuable when exploring situation awareness. Video playback can demonstrate how people react as more information becomes available, or highlight moments of task fixation. This can prompt a useful discussion around the role of communication in developing team situation awareness.

The impact of leadership and communication style can also be demonstrated. It is common for people to feel anxious during simulated practice, and video can be used to show how they remained outwardly controlled. Similarly, if a team leader issues instructions that are untargeted or vague, the team's response might be highlighted and reflected upon.

How are non-technical skills assessed?

A challenge in the assessment of NTS is that they are '*essential to learn, [but] difficult to measure*' (Zausig et al., 2009). Their use in formative assessment is straightforward. Rating systems of NTS are best when they include behavioural descriptors that can be used in observation and feedback. These are based on specific, observable behaviours that offer indicators of internal processes, and work well with debriefing techniques such as advocacy with inquiry.

For example, imagine you are the lead instructor running a simulation in which a patient with difficult IV access has been brought into the Emergency Department after an opioid overdose. One of the learning objectives is for the candidate to lead decision making in relation to failed IV access. Observable behaviours you could look for that link to decision making are:

Observable behaviours

- Did the candidate verbalise the options available? Did you hear them mention repeating attempts at peripheral cannulation? Did they ask for an intraosseous needle, or perhaps even central venous access?
- Once they had a list of options, did they consider any risks or benefits associated with each?
- How did they communicate the decision to their team, and how did they measure the success of their choice?

These questions capture different aspects of decision making. Candidates might run through much of this internally but encouraging them to verbalise is useful both for the candidate and the group. Therefore, you as the instructor can facilitate this with questions such as '*What are the options for IV access in this patient*', '*Why have you chosen this specific option for your patient?*' or

'*How will you know if this has worked?*' Some of these questions may sit more comfortably within a brief 'time-out' or in the debrief when there is space to explore the candidates' mental models without breaking the flow of the simulation.

Using NTS systems for summative assessment is, however, more challenging. Differences between rating systems mean agreement must be reached in advance about which is most appropriate for a given assessment. The chosen system must then be tested for its validity and reliability. Calibrating examiners to ensure that they give comparable ratings is difficult (Higham et al., 2023), so validation of assessments is a complex and time-consuming exercise.

To make NTS assessment as robust as possible, matrices are commonly used to support instructors in teaching and assessing NTS. Matrices usually include a series of behavioural descriptors linked to the NTS performance expected of the candidate. This gives the instructor clear, concrete examples to look for when they perform their assessment. The example below is an extract from the NTS matrix used on the Advanced Life Support (ALS) re-certification course.

NTS	NTS actions	Achieved	Not achieved
Decision making	Recognise there may be multiple treatment options, and choose the most appropriate. Re-assess the impact of treatment decisions made Scenario example(s): *reassessment patency of vascular access after interventions*		

Non-technical skills for teams

In the rest of this chapter we will consider a number of specific areas that are relevant to teaching on a life support course:

- Directed communication
- Read back
- Closed loops
- Decision review

Sometimes you may wish to draw attention to a non-technical skill during a simulation, but more often you will decide to raise it as a discussion point during the debrief. It can then be helpful to point the team towards enacting the points raised in their next group practice.

A number of life support courses deliberately give teams time to plan their activities before the casualty arrives, a technique called 'snap briefing'. This might only take a minute or two, but helps them remember to allocate roles, allows for anticipation of difficulties and can permit the development of contingency plans. This technique can be combined with 'sit-reps', or 'situation reports', where the team come back together for brief updates. An example might be of a trauma team who perform a snap brief before the arrival of their patient, followed by sit-reps after their primary and secondary surveys. These techniques allow for the exchange of information (situation awareness and team working), as well as identifying priorities (task management), team members who are task overloaded (task management) or reviewing patient progress after initial treatment (situation awareness and decision making).

Many of the specific techniques available relate to communication. Some well-recognised methods of sharing information in an emergency are SBAR or ISBARD (Chapter 6). Like the structure offered by ABCDE when assessing a patient, using these models helps to standardise the process.

Directed communication

When sharing information or instructions it is important to employ 'directed communication'. Put simply, directed communication is a message that is addressed at a clear target. Usually this means using a person's name, but can mean using their role if their name is unknown. There are two reasons why this technique is valuable.

The first relates to a problem called the 'diffusion of responsibility'. If an untargeted instruction is offered to a group, for example '*Can someone get me the intra-osseous equipment*', then each member of the team will assume that someone else will perform the task. The larger the group the less likely it is that someone will step forward. On the other hand, if someone's name is attached to the task ('*Paul, can you get me intra-osseous equipment*') it becomes a responsibility of that specific individual. The team leader also has the advantage of knowing with whom to check whether the task was completed.

The second reason for using someone's name in directed communication relates to how the brain processes auditory information. Environmental sounds are continuously (albeit subconsciously) monitored. The likelihood of information passing from the subconscious to the conscious mind depends on several factors. As noted previously, the amount of cognitive capacity a person has at a given time is crucial, but also personal relevance (or salience) is important. Fortunately, a person's name enjoys privileged processing in the brain, and even when under pressure is much more likely to survive the passage to consciousness than other, less personal, triggers. This is something called the 'cocktail party effect' (Wood and Cowan, 1995).

It may also be useful when using directed communication to ask the person whether they have the skills or knowledge to perform the task. '*Amir, please insert a tracheal tube*' may lead the recipient of that instruction to work outside their sphere of competence as they do not want to 'upset' the team leader by refusing. '*Amir, do you have the skill to intubate in this situation?*' immediately ascertains the stated skill level of that individual and assigns clear ownership of that task if the answer is affirmative.

Read back

Sending a message requires more than simply speaking. To be effective, a message must be composed, targeted at the correct recipient using directed communication and received correctly by the intended target.

Read back is a technique by which correct receipt can be confirmed. It requires any safety-critical message to be repeated aloud by the receiver. This act confirms two important details. Firstly, it demonstrates the intended team member has received the message, and secondly that the content of the message is accurate.

This technique is useful not just for communication within a team, but also when communicating with colleagues in other departments. Read back techniques can almost entirely eliminate communication errors between laboratory and ward (Barenfanger et al., 2004), it is therefore worth encouraging learners on provider courses to be meticulous in practising this technique.

Closed loop communication

Knowing that an instruction has been correctly received is obviously essential, but is often not the final objective of the team leader. The team leader's intention is usually to prompt an action, so the final step in effective communication must be to ensure that the instruction has been completed. It is good practice for the team member to report back when they have completed their task, but of course they must time this confirmation for a moment when the team leader is ready to hear it. Receiving this confirmation is 'closing the loop'. If the team member gets distracted and does not check back, then the team leader should be encouraged to prompt them for a status update if they do not automatically do so.

When teaching this on a provider course it is important that instructors do not pre-empt team members by magically making interventions happen, or contracting time too much. Encouraging the team to talk to each other rather than the instructor dominating, leads to more effective learning.

Decision review

Decision making depends on correct situation awareness, but even with perfect awareness there is a risk of faulty decisions. A series of cognitive biases can misdirect teams' choices, especially in time-pressured scenarios.

The ability to make safe decisions is degraded at times of high workload, and this is when biasing effects can be significant. It is beyond the scope of this book to discuss the many cognitive biases that we are prone to, so we will give two brief examples. Confirmation bias occurs when someone only seeks information that aligns with, rather than challenges, their preconceptions. Anchoring bias represents a cognitive error in which all subsequent information is viewed through the prism of the earliest information encountered. Research has shown that this even happens when the initial information is entirely irrelevant (Tversky and Kahneman, 1974).

Teams should build into their work a few moments where they can come together, update their situation awareness and review the decisions they have made. The potential hazards inherent in both of these biases can be limited by teaching team members to deliberately share alternative perspectives. In emergency situations, teams often resist pausing to review choices, but taking a short time out can in fact make their responses more efficient by reducing time wasted on unnecessary or low-priority tasks. On life support courses teams can be encouraged to take mini time-outs to re-evaluate, seek wider views and consider potential options.

Summary and learning

Non-technical skills are vital for good team performance, and ultimately, for providing good patient care.

These are skills that can be described, observed, and taught successfully on provider courses.

Helping people recognise innate limitations in human performance can reinforce the value of good team working.

Simple, easy-to-teach techniques help to get the best out of teams even when their membership is fluid.

CHAPTER 13

The wider role of the instructor

Introduction

You probably became an instructor for a number of reasons: because you enjoy teaching; because your job has a teaching commitment built into it; or because it is part of your career plan. Most instructors find that teaching helps them increase and/or maintain their own knowledge and motivation. They also find being an instructor hugely enjoyable because of the entry into a teaching community with equally dedicated clinicians.

Learning outcomes

This chapter will enable you to:

- Describe the essential qualities of an instructor
- Explore some of the differences between coaching and mentorship
- Develop an approach to mentoring that supports learning
- Support your fellow instructors

Pocket Guide to Teaching for Clinical Instructors, Fourth Edition.
Edited by Kate Denning, Kevin Mackie and Alan Charters, Andrew Lockey.
© 2025 John Wiley & Sons Ltd. Published 2025 by John Wiley & Sons Ltd.

What makes a good instructor?

Good instructors have a strong foundation of knowledge and skills that allows them to become (or at least aspire to be) role models for learners. The building blocks for this have been described by Hesketh et al. (2001) in four levels.

Level 1: clinical credibility

Instructor performance is based on the knowledge, skills and experience that each individual instructor brings to the role. You also need to demonstrate:

- Clinical application of the theoretical content from the provider course
- Understanding of the clinical context
- Knowledge and credibility

Level 2: expertise in teaching and learning methods

Good instructors make learning relevant, meaningful and fun, with all sessions thoroughly prepared. They provide the best conditions for effective learning, where candidates become active participants in the process. In order to achieve this, they must be competent in methods of teaching and in understanding how to apply these methods to facilitate candidate learning.

Level 3: in-role self-awareness

Through being aware of yourself and of your learners' needs and abilities, you can bring to the learning experience a dynamic quality that adds value to the basic facts. A key attribute is the ability to gauge the individual needs and strengths of each learner. A grasp of the principles outlined in this book, together with good interpersonal skills and a reflective attitude in the learning environment, enables instructors to provide appropriate, calibrated teaching, feedback and support. If you are aware of your own biases and barriers to learning, you can more easily relate to your learners and help them identify any of their own barriers.

Level 4: role model

Experienced instructors will tell you that they themselves learn something new from each course they attend. Their ability to reflect and learn adds to their credibility as an instructor. Learning has been described as a journey not a destination. Recording this journey is encouraged and can be achieved by maintaining a professional portfolio, where experiences gained can be maximised through review and reflection.

Supporting learning on life support courses

Most life support courses allocate 'mentors' to 'mentees' and allow time in the programme for that relationship to develop. In some countries the terms 'mentor' and 'mentee' have been modified to fit cultural norms. However, whatever words we use, formal or informal support of candidates allows us to get to know them better and see if they identify any individual or personal factors that may influence their learning. Mentoring or supporting learning provides the opportunity to find out more about the particular needs of individuals and think about inclusion and diversity, as discussed in Chapter 2.

Some courses may allow for an online meeting with candidates prior to the course, because initial in-course meetings may be less productive if mentors have had no prior contact with their mentees. This is where instructor responsibilities, supporting learning in the wider context, become clear. The instructor who has to leave early, or is late in arriving, will not be in a position to offer professional mentorship and risks losing credibility. A good course timetable will arrange for mentors to be grouped together, having contact with their mentees at the beginning and end of each day and during informal contact – at refreshment breaks and lunchtime, for instance. In addition, important information about a candidate's performance may only become evident at the faculty meeting, after the course has dispersed for the day. Mentors must ensure that they provide relevant feedback to their mentees before commencement of the following day's course.

Mentorship offers an opportunity for us to:

- Identify any specific learning needs
- Consider any extenuating circumstances
- Explore remediation options
- Acknowledge achievements

The key outcome of mentorship should be better understanding of the candidates. Mentors can: allay fears or anxieties; offer a safe space for additional questions; facilitate repeated practice of specific skills; reinforce key learning outcomes; and clearly state assessment decisions.

Mentor or learning support meetings should be structured to give time for group support as well as the all-important individual support. It is vital that candidates are given the *opportunity* to discuss their individual needs away from the group and that this is seen as being a programmed element and not reserved only for a candidate who is struggling.

Adopting an approach that focuses on the learner and is more aligned to coaching may help. We outline here some of the values, beliefs and differences in questions you may ask that are more congruent with a coaching approach.

Values and beliefs

You may find the two acronyms OUR CHOICE and SAFER helpful as they represent two key aspects of supporting learning. OUR CHOICE shows that it is up to us how and what we learn, whilst SAFER reminds us that at all times our learners should feel they are in a psychologically safe environment.

Values (for ourselves)	Beliefs (learning should be)
Open mindedness	**S**elf-directed
Understanding	**A**utonomous
Reliability	**F**orming new mental models to inform new behaviours
	Evaluating own learning
Curiosity	**R**eflective and **R**esourceful
Humility and **H**onesty	
Optimism	
Integrity	
Commitment	
Enthusiasm	

(Adapted from Lawrence, 2022)

It is helpful for instructors to remember how they felt as learners on a provider course; to reflect on our moments of defensiveness and 'moments of enlightenment' (the 'a-ha' moments). What was it that empowered us? What was it that limited us?

When learners experience feedback, it has the potential to provide a rich basis for self-reflection. Rather than feeling threatened when our mistakes are identified, we need to see them as an opportunity to learn and grow. Empathy as a mentor is about recalling how it *felt* as a candidate on a provider course, without letting our personal experience dominate the learners' experience. Our feelings are often affected by the way interactions are managed and by the language used. Consider the examples of statements versus open questions in Figure 13.1.

Statements	Open questions
Let's agree your objectives	What outcomes would you like to set for yourself?
You may want to consider changing the way you managed that scenario	What strategies have you used in previous experiences to overcome challenges you face?
I think you should be considering this course of action next	What are your priorities in ensuring you progress as an instructor?
If you research this author you will get more background information	Where do you feel the challenges are for you going forwards?

Figure 13.1 Statements versus open questions

It is particularly important to develop a bond with learners, although the transient nature of the relationship can make this a challenge. It will be your role as a mentor to follow up and support your learner, finding out what they need from the faculty, the course and their colleagues to be able to feel psychologically safe enough to benefit from the course.

Difficult conversations

Mentors may need to have difficult conversations with their mentees when concerns have been raised by the faculty about their knowledge, skills or attitude.

It is important to:

- Discover the learner's perspective on the apparent challenges the faculty are noticing
- Listen actively and provide a safe environment for the candidate to disclose their own concerns
- Have an honest conversation of relevant concerns that the faculty may have raised
- Avoid making assumptions about the learner's motives

- Support the learner's approach to their own development
- Inquire what the learner needs from the faculty in order to progress
- Be honest and straightforward when communicating assessment decisions

When managing difficult conversations about learner progress, such as telling them that they are not meeting the assessment criteria, it is advisable not to do this in isolation. We should consider who is invited to join the conversation. As instructors we often feel that we need support, but candidates themselves also need support. Ideally the mentor acts as a critical friend and offers continuity, but the candidate may also choose to have a colleague or peer with them. The course director or educator may also need to be present, but we should be careful not to overwhelm the candidate with the presence of too many people.

When mentoring candidates we need to create conditions in which they can also share their concerns with us. Very occasionally learners feel that they have been treated unfairly, or have been humiliated in front of their peers. As a mentor in this situation you have a difficult role to play. Invariably the problem arises out of a perception imbalance. Instructors do not set out to belittle or destroy learners, but this is sometimes how the learner perceives the situation. Whatever their feelings, they are valid, and unless we 'hear' them, the candidate will struggle to move on.

Providing structure to support learners

There may be some advantages to having clear aims for mentor or learner support meetings. These usually fall into three categories: initial meeting, progress meetings and assessment decision meetings.

Initial meeting

The first meeting should allow you to get to know your candidates and their own particular learning needs. Learners may say that they feel underprepared for the course: this is an opportunity to see how much of the pre-course information they have absorbed and to make sure they understand what is expected of them. An unprepared candidate may need significant support, but this should not be to the detriment of other learners. Pre-course materials emphasise the need for learners to prepare for the course, but it is extremely common for candidates to arrive inadequately prepared either through lack of time or misunderstanding the specific preparation they should have done.

If candidates have not let the course centre know about specific learning needs prior to the course, then this is a good time to ask if there are any. You may recall in Chapter 2 that reference was made on several occasions to asking the candidate what accommodations they need rather than making assumptions about what will help them. This initial mentor meeting is a chance for learners to share with the rest of the group and the instructors the kind of strategies and accommodations that they find helpful. If the whole group is part of the discussion, then the peer group can help support each other more effectively.

Progress meetings

These offer opportunities to check on progress and clarify any points that may help the learners. Sometime it is helpful to review any feedback they have received and ask them to reflect on these comments to find their own way of negotiating towards a successful completion of the course.

Assessment decision meetings

There are times within a course when it is essential to ensure that any assessment decisions are clearly articulated to the learners. This should occur in the debrief or summary of every teaching session, but you will sometimes find that there is a break down in transmission and reception of key messages, or that your mentee needs more support in understanding the assessment decision.

Instructor responsibilities

Regulations and requirements

Each course has a code of conduct and regulations for developing and maintaining instructor status. It is important to familiarise yourself with those that apply.

Attending faculty meetings

On many courses there are faculty meetings at the beginning of the course and at the end of each day. The initial meeting is a forum for all instructors to meet since often they may not know each other and have probably not all taught together before. The course director and the course coordinator can introduce instructors to each other, discuss the layout of the teaching environment, note any last minute changes to the programme and discuss the approach to any contentious areas that are being addressed in the curriculum.

The initial meeting also provides an opportunity to ensure that all instructors are prepared for the day ahead. Communicating with your fellow instructors is crucial to running an educationally sound teaching station. You should agree which part of the session each of you will undertake: who will open and close the session; who will facilitate the debrief; and how you will ensure that you foster a truly learner-centred approach. You can also discuss documentation and your approach to good time-keeping.

Faculty meetings at the end of the day tend to focus more on the candidates themselves, although any logistical or controversial issues that have arisen during the day may be discussed and rectified. The main aim of the discussion is to identify those candidates who need help and to formulate a plan to deliver this. This is also an opportunity to point out any candidate who has potential to be an instructor. Early identification of these qualities, and a conversation with the candidates involved, will help develop those qualities, assuming that to be the mutually desired outcome.

At the final faculty meeting, any formative and summative assessment decisions are discussed and agreed. Generally speaking the options are: learners may pass; they may be informed that they will need to retest in a particular area; or it may be recommended that they repeat the course in its entirety.

Supporting other instructors

Showing support for your fellow instructors is a vital part of the role, and you can achieve this by:

- Sitting at the back of the teaching space as moral support, and role modelling your interest
- Being an active participant with regards to teaching and assessment
- Providing feedback and support to discuss how a session went
- Being able to support fellow faculty with challenging questions if invited
- Guiding and supporting instructor candidates

Summary and learning

As an instructor you will be able to contribute to your colleagues' learning and development and help to provide a safer environment for your patients.

An important part of your role in supporting learning is recognising and valuing the individual needs of your candidates.

Providing some structure and content for learning support meetings is helpful for both instructors and candidates.

Being an instructor will provide you with an opportunity to continue to grow and learn as a teacher and facilitator of learning.

Many people find that, although the role of an instructor is demanding, it is a hugely enjoyable, rewarding and sociable activity.

References and further reading

Chapter 1

Bahrick H and Hall L (2005) The importance of retrieval failures to long-term retention: a metacognitive explanation of the spacing effect. *Journal of Memory and Language* 52, 566–577.

Bloom BS (1956) *Taxonomy of Educational Objectives. Handbook 1: The cognitive domain*. David McKay, New York.

Brown PC, Roediger III, HL and McDaniel MA (2014) *Make it Stick: The science of successful learning*. Belknap Press, Cambridge, MA.

Bryan J (2021) *Say my name: the importance of correct terms, titles and pronunciation*. Times Higher Education: Campus. https://www.timeshighereducation. com/campus/say-my-name-importance-correct-terms-titles-and-pronunciation (last accessed June 2024).

Chen L, Lin T and Tang S (2021) A qualitative exploration of nursing undergraduates' perceptions towards scaffolding in the flipped classroom of the Fundamental Nursing Practice Course: a qualitative study. *BMC Family Practice* 22, 245.

Chickering AW and Gamson ZF (1987) Seven principles for good teaching in undergraduate education. *AAHE Bulletin* 39, 3–7.

Pocket Guide to Teaching for Clinical Instructors, Fourth Edition.
Edited by Kate Denning, Kevin Mackie and Alan Charters, Andrew Lockey.
© 2025 John Wiley & Sons Ltd. Published 2025 by John Wiley & Sons Ltd.

Davis M and Denning K (2018) Listening through the learning conversation: a thought-provoking intervention. *MedEdPublish* 7, 199.

De Castro LT, Coriolano AM, Burckart K et al. (2022) Rapid-cycle deliberate practice versus after-event debriefing clinical simulation in cardiopulmonary resuscitation: a cluster randomized trial. *Advances in Simulation (London)* 7, 43.

Ericsson A, Krampe R and Tesch-Romer C (1993) The role of deliberate practice in the acquisition of expert performance. *Psychological Review* 100, 363–406.

Goleman D (1995) *Emotional Intelligence: Why it can matter more than IQ*. Bloomsbury Publishing, London.

Knowles M (1984) *The Adult Learner: A neglected species*, 3rd edn. Gulf Publishing, Houston.

Kolb D (1984) *Experiential Learning*. Prentice Hall, Englewood Cliffs.

Kornell N and Bjork R (2008) Learning concepts and strategies: is spacing the "enemy of induction"? *Psychological Science* 19, 582–592.

Kruger J and Dunning D (1999) Unskilled and unaware of it: how difficulties in recognizing one's own incompetence lead to inflated self-assessments. *Journal of Personality and Social Psychology* 77, 1121–1134.

Lockey A, Conaghan P, Bland A and Astin F (2021) Educational theory and its application to advanced life support courses: a narrative review. *Resuscitation Plus* 5, 100053.

Marshall S (2020) *A Handbook for Teaching and Learning in Higher Education: Enhancing academic practice*, 5th edn. Routledge, Taylor & Francis, London.

Maslow A (1971) *The Farther Reaches of Human Nature*. Viking Press, New York.

Mortiboys A (2012) *Teaching with Emotional Intelligence: A step by step guide for higher and further education professionals*, 2nd edn. Routledge, Abingdon.

Race P (2020) *The Lecturers Toolkit*, 5th edn. Routledge, London.

Ryan RM and Deci EL (2020) Intrinsic and extrinsic motivation form a self-determination theory perspective: definitions, theory, practices, and future directions. *Contemporary Educational Psychology* 61, article 101860.

Schon D (1987) *Educating the Reflective Practitioner: Toward a new design for teaching and learning in the professions*. Jossey Bass, San Francisco.

Syed M (2011) *Bounce: The myth of talent and the power of practice*. Fourth Estate, London.

Chapter 2

Espaillat A, Panna DK, Goede DL, Gurka MJ, Novak MA and Zaidi Z (2019) An exploratory study on microaggressions in medical school: what are they and why should we care? *Perspectives on Medical Education* 8, 143–151

Holley LC and Steiner S (2005) Safe space: student perspectives on classroom environment. *Journal of Social Work Education* 41, 49–64.

McKinsey & Company (2020) *Diversity wins. How inclusion matters*. https://www.mckinsey.com/~/media/McKinsey/Featured%20Insights/Diversity%20and%20Inclusion/Diversity%20wins%20How%20inclusion%20matters/Diversity-wins-How-inclusion-matters-vF.pdf (last accessed June 2024).

Sue DW (2010) *Microaggressions in Everyday Life: Race, gender, and sexual orientation*. John Wiley & Sons, Hoboken.

UNESCO International Bureau of Education (2016) *Training Tools for Curriculum Development. Reaching out to all learners: a resource pack for supporting inclusive education*. UNESCO. https://unesdoc.unesco.org/ark:/48223/pf0000243279 (last accessed June 2024).

Chapter 3

Merriam SB and Brockett RG (2007) *The Profession and Practice of Adult Education: An introduction*. Jossey-Bass, San Francisco.

Spencer B (2006) *The Purposes of Adult Education: A short introduction*, 2nd edn. Toronto: Thompson Educational Publishing, Toronto.

Chapter 4

Bion WR (1952) Group dynamics: a re-view. *International Journal of Psycho-Analysis* 33, 235–247.

Bion WR (1967) *Second Thoughts*. W. Heinemann Medical Books, London.

Brookfield S (1993) Through the lens of learning: how the visceral experience of learning reframes teaching. In: Boud D, Cohen R and Walker D (eds) *Using Experience for Learning*. SHRE/Open University, Buckingham.

Burgess A, van Diggele C, Roberts C and Mellis C (2020) Facilitating small group learning in the health professions. *BMC Med Educ* 20 (Suppl. 2), 457.

Jacques D (2015) *Small Group Teaching*, 2nd edn. Oxford Brookes University, Oxford.

Tuckman BW and Jensen MC (1977) Stages of small group development revisited. *Group and Organizational Studies* 2, 419–427.

Chapter 5

Breckwoldt J, Cheng A, Laurisden KG, Lockey A, Yeung J and Greif R (2023) Stepwise approach to skills teaching in resuscitation: a systematic review. *Resuscitation Plus* 16, 100457.

Brown PC, Roediger III, HL and McDaniel MA (2014) *Make it Stick: The science of successful learning*. Belknap Press, Cambridge, MA.

Bullock I (2000) Skill acquisition in resuscitation. *Resuscitation* 45, 139–143.

DeBourgh GA (2011) Psychomotor skills acquisition of novice learners. A case for contextual learning. *Nurse Education* 36, 144–149.

Ericsson KA, Krampe RT and Tesch-Römer C (1993). The role of deliberate practice in the acquisition of expert performance. *Psychological Review* 100, 363–406.

Fitts PM and Posner MI (1967) *Human Performance*. Brooks-Cole, Belmont.

Nicholls D, Sweeta L, Mullera A and Hyettc J (2016) Teaching psychomotor skills in the twenty-first century: revisiting and reviewing instructional approaches through the lens of contemporary literature. *Medical Teacher* 38, 1056–1063.

Patocka C, Khan F, Dubrovsky AS, Brody D, Bank I and Bhanji F (2015) Pediatric resuscitation training – instruction all at once or spaced over time? *Resuscitation* 88, 6–11.

Simpson EJ (1972) *The Classification of Educational Objectives in the Psychomotor Domain*, Vol. 3. Gryphon House, Washington.

Walker M and Peyton R (1998) Teaching in theatre. In: Peyton JWR (ed) *Teaching and Learning in Medical Practice*. Manticore Publishing Europe, Rickmansworth, pp. 171–180.

Chapter 6

Briceño E (2016) *How to get better at the things you care about*. TEDx. https://www.ted.com/talks/eduardo_briceno_how_to_get_better_at_the_things_you_care_about?language=en (last accessed June 2024).

Buchanan DA and Huczynski A (2013) *Organizational Behaviour*, 8th edn. Pearson Education, Harlow.

Rudolph JW, Raemer DB and Simon R (2014) Establishing a safe container for learning simulation. *Society for Simulation in Healthcare* 9, 339–349.

Chapter 7

Bravata DM, Madhusudhan DK, Boroff M and Cokley KO (2020) Commentary: prevalence, predictors, and treatment of imposter syndrome: a systematic review. *Journal of Mental Health and Clinical Psychology* 4, 12–16.

Dweck C (2006) *Mindset: The new psychology of success*. Ballantine Books, New York.

Dweck C (2016) *What having a growth mindset actually means*. Harvard Business Review. https://hbr.org/2016/01/what-having-a-growth-mindset-actually-means (last accessed June 2024).

Gilbert P (2009) *The Compassionate Mind: A new approach to life challenges*. Constable and Robinson, London.

Irons C and Beaumont E (2017) *The Compassionate Mind Workbook: A step-by-step guide to developing your compassionate self*. Robinson, London.

Mullangi S and Jagsi R (2019) Imposter syndrome: treat the cause, not the symptom. *JAMA*, 322(5), 403–404.

Tulshyan R and Burey JA (2021) *Stop telling women they have imposter syndrome*. Harvard Business Review. https://hbr.org/2021/02/stop-telling-women-they-have-imposter-syndrome (last accesssed June 2024).

Van der Kolk B (2014) *The Body Keeps the Score: Mind, brain and body in the transformation of trauma*. Penguin, London.

Welford M (2016) *Compassion Focussed Therapy for Dummies*. John Wiley & Sons, Chichester.

Chapter 8

Argyris C, Putnam R and Smith D. *Action Science*. Jossey-Bass, San Francisco.

Askew S and Lodge C (2000) Gifts, ping-pong and loops – linking feedback and learning. In: Askew S, ed. *Feedback for Learning*. Routledge, London, pp. 1–17.

Carr S (2006) The foundation programme assessment tools: an opportunity to enhance feedback to trainees? *Postgraduate Medical Journal* 82, 576–579.

Chowdhury R and Kalu G (2006) Learning to give feedback in medical education. *Obstetrician and Gynaecologist* 6, 243–247.

Davis M and Denning K. (2018) Listening through the learning conversation: a thought provoking intervention. *MedEdPublish* 7, 199.

Juwah C, McFarlane-Dick D, Matthew R, Nicol D, Ross D and Smith B (2004) *Enhancing Student Learning Through Effective Formative Feedback*. Higher Education Academy Generic Centre.

Rudolph J, Simon R, Rivard P, Dufresne R and Raemer D (2007) Debriefing with good judgment: combining rigorous feedback with genuine inquiry. *Anaesthesiology Clinics* 25, 361–376.

Saunders S and Gowing R (1999) Learning from the learning conversation: benefits and problems in developing a process to improve workplace performance. In: Summary of Presentation at the 3rd International Conference 'Researching Vocational Education and Training', 14–16 July 1999, Bolton Institute.

Sawyer T, Eppich W, Brett-Fleegler M, Grant V and Cheng A (2016) More than one way to debrief: a critical review of healthcare simulation debriefing methods. *Simulation in Healthcare* 11, 209–217.

Chapter 9

Miller G (1990) The assessment of clinical skills/competence/performance. *Academic Medicine* 65 (Suppl.), S63–S67.

Schut S, Driessen E, van Tartwijk J, van der Vleuten C and Heeneman S (2018) Stakes in the eye of the beholder: an international study of learners' perceptions within programmatic assessment. *Medical Education* 52, 654–663.

Van der Vluten C and Schuwirth L (2005) Assessing professional competence: from methods to programmes. *Medical Education* 39, 309–317.

Westwood OMR and Griffin A (eds) (2013) *How to Assess Students and Trainees in Medicine and Health*. Wiley-Blackwell, Oxford.

Wilkinson T, Frampton C, Thompson-Fawcett M and Egan T (2003) Objectivity in objective structured clinical examinations: checklists are no substitute for examiner commitment. *Academic Medicine* 78, 219–223.

Chapter 10

Bloom B, Englehart M, Furst E, Hill W and Krathwohl D (1956) *Taxonomy of Educational Objectives: The classification of educational goals. Handbook I: Cognitive domain.* Longmans, Green, New York and Toronto.

Cantillon P, Wood D and Yardley S (2017) *ABC of Learning and Teaching in Medicine*, 3rd edn. BMJ Books, Wiley, Oxford.

Sellappah S, Hussey T, Blackmore AM and McMurray A (1998) The use of questioning strategies by clinical teachers. *Journal of Advanced Nursing* 28, 142–148.

Chapter 11

Elgohary M, Palazzo FS, Breckwoldt J et al. (2022) Blended learning for accredited life support courses – a systematic review on behalf of the EIT Task Force of ILCOR. *Resuscitation Plus* 10, 100240.

Lockey AS, Bland A, Stephenson J, Bray J and Astin F (2022) Blended learning in healthcare education: an overview and overarching meta-analysis of systematic reviews. *Journal of Continuing Education in the Health Professions* 42, 256–264.

Quinn CN (2012) *The Mobile Academy: m-learning for higher education.* Jossey-Bass, San Francisco.

Chapter 12

Arora S, Miskovic D, Hull L et al. (2011) Self vs expert assessment of technical and non-technical skills in high fidelity simulation. *American Journal of Surgery* 202, 500–506.

Barenfanger J, Sautter RL, Lang DL, Collins SM, Hacek DM and Peterson LR (2004) Improving patient safety by repeating (read-back) telephone reports of critical information. *American Journal of Clinical Pathology* 121, 801–803.

Frerk C, Mitchell VS, Mcnarry AF et al. (2015) Difficult Airway Society 2015 guidelines for management of unanticipated difficult intubation in adults. *British Journal of Anaesthesia* 115, 827–848.

Glavin RJ (2011) Human performance limitations (communication, stress, prospective memory and fatigue). *Best Practice and Research Clinical Anaesthesiology* 25, 193–206.

Higham H, Greig P, Crabtree N, Hadjipavlou G, Young D and Vincent C (2023) A study of validity and usability evidence for non-technical skills assessment tools in simulated adult resuscitation scenarios. *BMC Medical Education* 23, 153.

Mussweiler T and Strack F (2006) Playing dice with criminal sentences: the influence of irrelevant anchors on experts' judicial decision making. *Personality and Social Psychology Bulletin* 32, 188–200.

Riem N, Boet S, Bould MD, Tavares W and Naik VN (2012) Do technical skills correlate with non-technical skills in crisis resource management: a simulation study. *British Journal of Anaesthesia* 109, 723–728.

Tversky A and Kahneman D (1974) Judgment under uncertainty: heuristics and biases. *Science* 185, 1124–1131.

Wood N and Cowan N (1995) The cocktail party phenomenon revisited: how frequent are attention shifts to one's name in an irrelevant auditory channel? *Journal of Experimental Psychology* 21, 255–260.

Zausig YA, Grube C, Boeker-Blum T et al. (2009) Inefficacy of simulator-based training on anaesthesiologists' non-technical skills. *Acta Anaesthesiologica Scandinavica* 53, 611–619.

Chapter 13

Hesketh E, Bagnall G, Buckley E et al. (2001) A frame-work for developing excellence as a clinical educator. *Medical Education* 35, 555–564.

Kline N (1999) *Time to Think: Listening to Ignite the Human Mind*. Cassell Illustrated, London.

Lawrence J (2022) RO Forum presentation. RCUK Conference, Birmingham, December 2022.

Index

A

adult learning
  andragogy, 13–14
  defined, 31
Advanced Paediatric Life
  Support (APLS), 73
advocacy with inquiry, 96,
  97, 146
andragogy, 13–14
arousal states, 72
assessment, 101–12
  continuous, 104, 107, 109
  formal, 104
  formative, 103, 104
  forms of, 108
  informal, 104
  principles, 105–9
  purpose of, 102–3
  summative, 103, 104, 107,
    109, 147
  teaching structure, 110–11
  types of, 103–4
assessment decisions
  communicating, 36, 37,
    109, 111, 159
  supporting, 106

assessment for/of learning,
  104
assessment materials, 34
associative stage of
  learning, 54, 55
auditory learning
  preference, 131
automatic stage of learning,
  54, 56

B

basic-assumption mode, 41
beliefs, 156–9
belonging, sense of, 18–19
blended learning, 127–35
  application in life support
    courses, 132–5
  potential benefits/
    limitations, 128–9
Bloom's taxonomy, 13, 45
body language, 48, 49
box breathing exercise, 82

C

candidate engagement,
  maximising, 50–2

Pocket Guide to Teaching for Clinical Instructors, Fourth Edition.
Edited by Kate Denning, Kevin Mackie and Alan Charters, Andrew Lockey.
© 2025 John Wiley & Sons Ltd. Published 2025 by John Wiley & Sons Ltd.

How to use your textbook

The anytime, anywhere textbook

Wiley E-Text

Your textbook comes with free access to a **Wiley E-Text: Powered by VitalSource** version – a digital version of this textbook which you own as soon as you download it.

Your **Wiley E-Text** allows you to:

Search: Save time by finding terms and topics instantly in your book, your notes, even your whole library (once you've downloaded more textbooks)

Note and highlight: Colour code, highlight and make digital notes right in the text so you can find them quickly and easily

Organize: Keep books, notes and class materials organized in folders inside the application

Share: Exchange notes and highlights with others

Upgrade: Your textbook can be transferred when you need to change or upgrade computers

The **Wiley E-Text** version will also allow you to copy and paste any photograph or illustration into assignments, presentations and your own notes.

Pocket Guide to Teaching for Clinical Instructors, Fourth Edition.
Edited by Kate Denning, Kevin Mackie and Alan Charters, Andrew Lockey.
© 2025 John Wiley & Sons Ltd. Published 2025 by John Wiley & Sons Ltd.

To access your Wiley E-Text:

- Find the redemption code on the inside front cover of this book and carefully scratch away the top coating of the label. Visit **http://www.vitalsource.com/downloads** to download the Bookshelf application to your computer, laptop, tablet or mobile device.
- If you have purchased this title as an e-book, access to your **Wiley E-Text** is available with proof of purchase within 90 days. Visit **http://support.wiley.com** and click on the 'Contact Support' tab.
- Open the Bookshelf application on your computer and register for an account.
- Follow the registration process and enter your redemption code to download your digital book.

The VitalSource Bookshelf can now be used to view your Wiley E-Text on iOS, Android and Kindle Fire!

- **For iOS:** Visit the app store to download the VitalSource Bookshelf: **http://bit.ly/17ib3XS**
- **For Android and Kindle Fire:** Visit the Google Play Market to download the VitalSource Bookshelf: **http://bit.ly/BSAAGP**

You can now sign in with the email address and password you used when you created your VitalSource Bookshelf Account

Full E-Text support for mobile devices is available at: **http://support.vitalsource.com**

Contributors to the first, second and third editions

Ian Bullock
London

Andrew Coleman
Northampton

Mick Colquhoun
Cardiff

Pat Conaghan
Manchester

Mike Davis
Blackpool

Kate Denning
Plymouth

Peter Driscoll
Manchester

David Gabbott
Bristol

Carl Gwinnutt
Manchester

Sue Hampshire
London

Bob Harris
London

Duncan Harris
London

Sara Harris
London

Jane Hatfield
Oxford

Gareth Holsgrove
Cambridge

Pauline Howard
Oxford

Melanie Humphreys
Wolverhampton

Lynn Jones
Manchester

Pocket Guide to Teaching for Clinical Instructors, Fourth Edition.
Edited by Kate Denning, Kevin Mackie and Alan Charters, Andrew Lockey.
© 2025 John Wiley & Sons Ltd. Published 2025 by John Wiley & Sons Ltd.

Andrew Lockey
Halifax

Kevin Mackie
Birmingham

Kevin Mackway-Jones
Manchester

Sarah Mitchell
London

Jerry Nolan
Oxford

Elizabeth Norris
Bath

Gavin Perkins
Birmingham

Russell Perkins
Manchester

Mike Walker
London

Terence Wardle
Chester

Celia Warlow
Northampton

Sue Wieteska
Manchester

Jonathan Wyllie
Middlesbrough

Jackie Younker
Bristol